T0162597

TOTAL HEALTH with the 5 ELEMENTS

QIGONG
FOR SELF-REFINEMENT

WRITTEN AND ILLUSTRATED BY
CHRIS SHELTON

COVER DESIGNED BY
JOSE ERNESTO PALACIOS

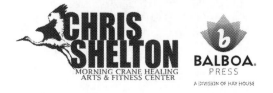

CHRIS SHELTON
MORNING CRANE HEALING
ARTS & FITNESS CENTER

BALBOA
PRESS
A DIVISION OF HAY HOUSE

Balboa Press books may be ordered through booksellers or by contacting:

Balboa Press
A Division of Hay House
1663 Liberty Drive
Bloomington, IN 47403
www.balboapress.com
1-(877) 407-4847

Printed in the United States of America.

Medical disclaimer

The meditations, practices and techniques described in this book are not to be used as an alternative or substitute for professional medical treatment. This book does not attempt to give any medical diagnosis of or recommendations for any human disease, ailment or condition. The author cannot be responsible for the results of any use or misuse of the information presented here.

For further information on the practices described here, or to register for a course, please visit www.MorningCrane.com. For further information about the author, please visit www.ChrisjShelton.com.

ISBN: 978-1-4525-7474-5 (sc)
ISBN: 978-1-4525-7472-1 (hc)
ISBN: 978-1-4525-7473-8 (e)

Library of Congress Control Number: 2013909464

Balboa Press rev. date: 6/14/2013

DEDICATION

This book is dedicated to my beautiful wife Parisa who makes my world turn; to Martha who transformed my notes and knowledge into a manuscript; to the countless friends and family who support my passions; and to my loyal students who make my work worthwhile. Thank you.

Table of Contents

FOREWORD.. xi

INTRODUCTION xiii

How to Use This Book xix

Chapter 1: FOUNDATIONS 1

    Centers of Energy: The Dan Tians...2

    Basic Guidelines for Practicing Qigong.....................................3

    The Three Regulations 4

    Wu Ji Posture 5

    White Pearl Meditation 6

Chapter 2: THE NATURE OF QI 9

    BODY AWAKENING EXERCISES... 11

    CENTER AND BALANCE MEDITATION.................................. 13

Chapter 3: THE MERIDIAN SYSTEM.. 15

    BRUSHING THE MERIDIANS 17

Chapter 4: YIN AND YANG OF THE ORGANS.............................21

    MASSAGING THE YANG ORGANS...23

Chapter 5: THE VESSELS AND GATES...25

    MICRO-COSMIC ORBIT MEDITATION.......................................27

Chapter 6: FIVE ELEMENTS IN DETAIL 31

    COLLECTING HEAVEN AND EARTH 33

Chapter 7: FIRE ELEMENT 35

    HEART CLEANSING EXERCISE 39

Chapter 8: EARTH ELEMENT 43

    EARTH ELEMENT IMBALANCE 44

    SPLEEN CLEANSING EXERCISE 46

Chapter 9: METAL ELEMENT 49

    LUNG CLEANSING EXERCISE 53

Chapter 10: WATER ELEMENT 55

    KIDNEY CLEANSING EXERCISE 61

Chapter 11: WOOD ELEMENT 65

    LIVER CLEANSING EXERCISE 68

Chapter 12: STAYING PRESENT 71

    SUGGESTED DAILY ROUTINES 72

    RENEWAL OF SPIRIT MEDITATION 74

Chapter 13: THE FIVE ELEMENT QUESTIONNAIRE 77

Chapter 14: FIRE ARCHETYPE 79

Chapter 15: EARTH ARCHETYPE 85

Chapter 16: METAL ARCHETYPE 89

Chapter 17: WATER ARCHETYPE 93

Chapter 18: WOOD ARCHETYPE 97

Chapter 19: THE EMOTIONAL COMPONENT 101

Chapter 20: CONCLUSION 107

APPENDICES 109

FIVE ELEMENT CHART 109

FIVE ELEMENT QUESTIONNAIRE 110

FIVE ELEMENT QUESTIONNAIRE ANSWERS 116

SELF-REFLECTION CHECKLIST 117

RECOMMENDED READING AND REFERENCES.................... 122

FOREWORD

I first heard about the amazing Chris Shelton from MMA superstar and actor, Cung Le. He told me that Chris was his Chinese energy specialist who used unusual and ancient methods to heal Cung's battle-worn body. Having had a 30 year history with martial arts myself, I was captivated by Cung's description of the treatments Chris had administered. I always felt that Western medicine had missed the key to overall health by treating the symptoms of illness rather than solving ailments at the root of origin. Chris had a holistic approach and had the advanced training to back up his methods of healing. This tattooed, fit, white guy from San Jose was "the real deal" and I needed to meet him in person.

As soon as we met, we instantaneously became great friends. In many ways our skill sets compliment each other, mine in perfecting the external body and his increasing the dynamic health of the internal energy systems. We complete each other professionally, yet it's Chris' personality which draws me and so many others to want to be around him. His genuine care for those suffering in pain and discomfort and his unwavering conviction to make a difference in people's lives by increasing the quality of their daily existence puts him in a league of selfless individuals that are rarely spotted in normal life. I am honored to call Chris a friend, a colleague, and someone who came to my rescue after a lower back injury left me limping in pain. Chris' treatments allowed the healing to come swiftly and effectively.

In this book you will learn practices that will slow down the aging process, prevent and eliminate disease, and increase your wellness and vitality. You will also learn your archetype, which relates to your constitution. There are tools in this book that will improve your mental and emotional well being. I trust that the direct application of these methods will enrich your life and expand your understanding of ways to look, feel, and live a better life. Enjoy the journey....

"Eric the Trainer"
Eric P. Fleishman
Hollywood Physique Expert
Los Angeles, CA
June 1, 2013

INTRODUCTION

This book describes the theories and practices of a Chinese exercise system known as "Qigong". "Qi" refers to the life force energy that emanates in all things material and non-material, and "gong" means work or skill. Doing the meditations and exercises described here will certainly give your Qi a workout, but you will finish feeling revitalized and refreshed, rather than worked-out exhausted. Each day of practice should bring greater and greater benefits, gradually refining your health and vitality—your fundamental nature—as one would refine ore into gold.

The book began as a collection of handouts for a course I teach. Here you will find both those handouts and the text of the accompanying lectures. Thus it can serve either as a complete self-study guide for anyone who would like to explore the effects of this ancient, extraordinary system, or as a reference for those who have taken my course. No special equipment required: The meditations and exercises are simple; you need only patience and perseverance to succeed.

The first section of the book (Chapters 1-12) focuses on Chinese theories of how the body functions, and teaches practices based on these theories. The Chinese see the body as an intricate network of energy pathways. Each pathway is associated with particular functions and organs, and each pathway can be influenced by particular movements, sounds, and even thoughts. Practicing the meditations and exercises described in this book, you can learn to stimulate and harmonize the vital energy in your own body. Examples of how these exercises have helped me and my clients are also included.

The second section of the book (Chapters 13-19) focuses on Five Element theory as it applies to people. The Five Elements are expressed in what people look like, as well as how they behave; they can be used to diagnose disease as well as enhance life. Emotions are a key component of health, so addressing emotional issues is absolutely critical in all that I teach and in my healing practice. Tools that I have found useful in restoring emotional balance are also briefly described.

The final chapter (Chapter 20) brings it all together. The Qigong practices, application of Five Element theory, and emotional work comprise an effective, comprehensive means of understanding your fundamental nature, of refining your Qi, and thereby of realizing your full potential as a human being.

Personal history

My path to Qigong started at age 17, after two heart attacks from drugs and a near-paralyzing back injury from a bad kick in Tae Kwon Do. It is no exaggeration to say that Qigong saved my life.

As a teenager I was rebellious and arrogant, with an explosive temper. My friends were doing drugs, so—hey, why not me too? I felt invincible—until I ended up in the emergency room from a drug overdose. Finally, it became clear that continuing on my present course would put me either in prison or the grave. I decided that taking up Tae Kwon Do would be my ticket to a new life. I trained hard, enjoying the vigorous and challenging exercise, until one night, during training for a tournament, I was accidentally kicked in the back. The blow left me almost paralyzed. For the first time in my life I experienced helplessness. I couldn't wipe myself in the bathroom or put on my own shoes and socks. From an x-ray of my back, a chiropractor confirmed what the Western doctors had told me: if I wasn't careful, the injury could paralyze me from the waist down. She referred me to a massage therapist who was also a martial artist. While he worked on me, he talked about Qi. As a 17-year old boy I was convinced that this Qi was some kind of hocus-pocus. My Tae Kwon Do instructors had talked about "Ki" but only in terms of the sound that you make at the moment you throw a punch or kick. What this massage therapist was describing seemed entirely different. He told me that, yes, Qi could be used for martial arts but it also could be used to heal.

Intrigued, impressed by his sincerity, and feeling better, I started taking Qigong classes. At that time, because of my years of drug use I had kidney problems, liver problems, sinusitis, and digestive problems. The digestive problems were so severe that an hour after eating I was nauseated; I survived on products like Tum's and Kaopectate. So I started Qigong, doing the guided meditations and gentle moving practices regularly, but without real dedication. I was really just going through the motions, as they say. Even so, after some time—perhaps six months or a year—I realized that all my health ailments had gone away. I was breathing easily, and I could eat without feeling sick to my stomach! Similarly, the other two women in the class, one with arthritis and the other with asthma, reported that their conditions had almost completely resolved by the end of the year.

As my internal organs recovered, so did my back. The Western doctors went from saying that I'd never be able to walk again to saying that I'd be able to walk but I'd never be able to train again. Then they said that I'd be able to train again, but I'd never be able to fight again. Proving them wrong, I competed in Kungfu and kickboxing tournaments two years ago at age 40.

What is Qi?

But even after recovering, even after experiencing the power of these deceptively simple exercises, I still didn't fully understand what Qi was or how this miracle had happened. All I knew was that there was something to it: somehow it worked. Now, after more than twenty years of practicing and working with Qi, I have more of an appreciation of what Qi is, and can offer the following description.

According to the Chinese, Qi is the energy that creates, infuses and sustains the universe. It is said to be present in inanimate objects, like rocks, as well as in living things like plants and animals, as well as in the subtle states of immaterial things like the air, light, sound and thought. There are different kinds of Qi.

If Qi is strong and coherent, life flourishes. Conversely, if Qi becomes stagnant, deficient or scatters, this opens the door for disease and, ultimately, for death. Qigong is a means of working with, cultivating, and developing your personal Qi. In other words, it is a method for maintaining your vital life force. It is not based on belief; you do not have to believe in it for it to work. The concept of Qi is at the heart of traditional Chinese medicine theory, and Qigong-type exercises are as old as the medicine itself. The fact that this medicine has been around more than 5000 years is in itself evidence that it works. History has shown that anything fake or false inevitably reveals its flaws over time, and is discarded. (I would like to add here, that to do Qigong; you do not have to wear fancy silk pajamas or a cloak.)

How does it work? According to Chinese medical theory, Qi flows in specific pathways in the body, called "meridians". Each meridian is associated with a particular organ; for the most part, the Chinese organs correspond to anatomical organs. In some sense, meridians can be compared to rivers, and the internal organs to lakes that are supplied and drained by the rivers. Thus, just as in nature, when not enough water flows in a river, the lake it feeds will dry out, adversely affecting the surrounding environment and all the related ecosystems. Conversely, when too much water flows, the lake will overflow its boundaries. Using this metaphor we can say that the purpose of Qigong is to balance and harmonize the rivers and lakes of the body so that they function at their peak capacity.

Beauty beyond the physical

According to Chinese medicine, the two leading causes of disease are negative emotions and diet. Diet and emotions influence the body differently, but ultimately interact. Diet supplies the physical substance from which the body continually recreates itself. Emotions, too, are a kind of diet because they determine the quality of the subtle energies of the body which control organ function. Based on observations made by doctors over centuries, Chinese medical theory posits that the internal organs store different negative emotions, and when these emotions are held or expressed inappropriately the proper function of the related organs is disrupted, sometimes causing fatal health problems. Different organs store different kinds of energy, and are damaged by excesses or deficiencies of these particular energies. The Chinese also understand that these internal organs are interrelated, such that a dysfunction of one can eventually lead to a dysfunction of another. Thus, in clinical practice, a doctor can work backward from the disease that is manifesting to the emotional toxins to find the true root of a condition.

Another aspect of emotional health is one's attitude toward aging and beauty. Aging is inevitable; we all must face decline in our physical faculties. So often nowadays we see people focusing on their external beauty, having surgery or liposuction and using techniques like Botox. Chinese medicine in general and Qigong in particular address this issue from two standpoints. First, it tackles the attitude. Why is a person so concerned about appearance? Is there fear? Hate? Exploring these questions can be very important. When your organs are in harmony, you will feel so good—enjoying your life, your family, and your passions—that you will not have time for such thoughts. Second, it asks you to reassess what beauty means. When your organs, including your skin, are functioning properly, not storing negative emotions or toxic digestive waste, you will radiate health—and beauty at any age.

Simple practices, profound results

To our Western mind, it seems incredible that these simple movements and meditations can have such profound effects. No surgery? Supplements? Drugs?? But it is true. You can experience this yourself. Indeed, one of the values of Qigong is that you gradually can become your own doctor. Doing these practices will put you in touch with your body in subtle ways. You will develop sensitivity, both to emotional and physical conditions in your body. Eventually you will be able to detect disease as it sets in. You will know the first signs of imbalance, and with the meditations and exercises described in this book, you will have tools to try to correct them.

If you have a hard time accepting the concept of Qi or the theories about how it works, then—just as I did in the beginning—ignore it all! Just do the exercises. Based on the successful experiences of countless generations of people who have used these exercises and passed them down to us, give them a try. Observe carefully. The body has its own wisdom as to how and when it heals. You may be surprised with what happens, and it may not happen as you expect. Simply practice consistently. Over time you will experience greater vitality, health and mental well-being.

The journey of a thousand miles begins with a single step. Take that step, and enjoy the journey!

Chris Shelton
May, 2013
Willow Glen, CA

How to Use This Book

If you are new to Chinese medical theories, I recommend that you start at the beginning and work through each chapter just as though you were taking my course. The information in each chapter corresponds to one lesson of my course; each builds on the previous. In particular, there are many terms and concepts that are specific to the Chinese; I have tried to explain each new term before I use it. While you may have a particular health concern that you are trying to address—arthritis, or high blood pressure, for example—the body is still a coherent whole system. What affects one system will affect the whole. By working through the book you will become acquainted with how the Chinese conceive of these body parts working together, and thus how affecting one will affect another. Thus when you address your issue (or those of your clients, if you are a health practitioner) you will also be aware of changes elsewhere in the body so that you can maintain overall good health.

If you are familiar with Chinese medical theories and perhaps other forms of Qigong, then you may be able to go directly to the sections that interest you. Nevertheless, I do recommend that you at least skim through the other sections, if only for review. Hopefully, you will find some new kernel of knowledge that will increase and deepen your understanding. In any case, remember that the body is a coherent whole, and we must keep the whole picture in mind as we work on one part of it.

For everyone, Chapter 12 gives suggestions for establishing a regular practice. Regularity is important; the body has rhythms just as the cosmos does. Patience and persistence are important because results may come slowly, especially at first. The more you practice the more quickly you will experience results; however, even more important than the amount of time you spend is the quality of that time. Your undistracted attention is absolutely critical. In the beginning you may be simply learning to say focused; that is good. As in any mindfulness training, keep trying, without disappointment or frustration, and your body will respond. Your Qi will flourish.

Chapter 1: FOUNDATIONS

People know when they are sick; they also know how they feel when they are well. This is a matter of awareness of what the Chinese call "Qi." The practice of Qigong (pronounced *chee-gung*) focuses on refining this awareness. Which part of the body is sick? What is wrong with the Qi? Is it stuck? Is there too much or too little? Through the meditations and exercises of Qigong, we can answer these questions—and learn how to remedy problems. By practicing them, we can experience and create vibrant health.

Just as we know in our bodies when something is not quite right, we can also feel differences in the weather, as well as in people, even before they speak. All of this awareness involves energy. The ancient Chinese devised a universal system to describe the various forms of energy, not only in the human body and in the weather, but also in space (in landscape and geography) and over time (in history and astrology). By understanding that everything in the cosmos is an expression of Qi, from the material to the insubstantial, one can glimpse the ultimate truth of the universe and come to a deep understanding for and appreciation of the natural world, including one's own true nature.

The core text of Chinese philosophy is the *I Ching,* or the *Book of Changes.* Its basic premise is that energy evolves from the unmanifested to the manifested realm. These manifestations may be broadly described as Yin and Yang. Beyond Yin and Yang, all manifestations may be more precisely (but still generally) described in terms of the Five Elements. Beyond that, there are the "ten thousand things," all of which are permutations of these broader concepts.

Health is an expression of the smooth flow of life-giving Qi in the body. Disease manifests when the flow of Qi is blocked or stagnant, or when there is too much or too little. Physical and mental exercise can clear blockages, dissolve stagnation, reduce excess, and supplement deficiency. I will use these terms "excess" and "deficient" often throughout this text because these are the terms used in Chinese medical theory. They describe conditions in which there is too much of something, i.e., when an organ is hyperactive, or when there is too little, i.e., the organ is weak or hypoactive.

In these chapters, we will learn how to interpret the signs and signals of the body in terms of these patterns and how to correct and improve the flow of Qi. That is the practice and purpose of Qigong. It can benefit you as well as your clients or patients if you are a health practitioner.

Centers of Energy: The Dan Tians

Three is a number often used to describe or to simplify the complexity of our human experience. In Christianity, the aspects of God are described as Father, Son, and Holy Ghost. In Chinese metaphysics, the components of the universe are described as Heaven, Earth, and Man. In the human body, Chinese medical theory sees three "Dan Tians" (pronounced *dahn tee-ens*), or energy centers, corresponding to the physical, emotional/mental, and spiritual aspects of a person's being. These vital energy centers are located along the midline of the body and store energy much the way batteries do.

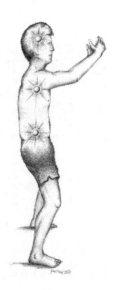

Upper

The Upper Dan Tian relates to our spiritual being. It roughly comprises the upper and posterior portions of the skull. In Western medicine, the

Upper Dan Tian corresponds to the central nervous system, which, through nerve impulses, controls the functions of all the organs.

Middle

The Middle Dan Tian relates to our mental/emotional state and is associated with the heart center in the middle of the chest.

Lower

The Lower Dan Tian relates to the physical aspect of our being and is located about an inch below the navel in the center of the body. This is the center most people refer to when they speak of "the Dan Tian." As all physical energy is stored and used from this region, we will refer to it often in our Qigong practice.

Basic Guidelines for Practicing Qigong

Practical Aspects

The goal of Qigong is to harmonize and develop your energy. If you do what you can to harmonize the physical aspects of the practice—your body and the environment—you will achieve your goal more quickly and to a much greater extent. When your body and mind are nourished, rested, calm, and relaxed, you will be in a natural state of equilibrium. Smooth flow of vigorous Qi will be expressed in your health and vitality.

Time and Place

1. Practice in a clean, well-ventilated place.

2. Practice at a time and in a place where you will not be disturbed.

3. Practice regularly—ideally in the same place at the same time.

4. Avoid eating meals thirty to sixty minutes before practice. At the

same time, do not practice when hungry. Your body should be comfortable and relaxed.

5. If you do heavy anaerobic exercise, such as weight lifting, on a day you do Qigong, be sure to stretch before and after to keep the meridians open.

Lifestyle

6. Get proper rest and sleep.

7. Avoid drinks that are ice cold.

8. Avoid drugs and alcohol.

9. Moderate your sexual activity.

10. Women: Stop practice during your monthly period, or, if you do practice, shift focus to the middle Dan Tian.

The Three Regulations

Breath

Breathing should be natural, slow, smooth, even, and deep. Allow the abdomen to relax so that it rises with each inhalation and falls with each exhalation. Do not use force. At the end of the exhalation, the body itself will initiate the inhalation. Always breathe through your nose.

Mind

Like the breathing, the mind should be relaxed. At the same time, it needs to be focused because visualization is used in most of the meditations, and later, the mind will be used to guide Qi. Balance relaxation with alert curiosity as to what is happening in your body and with firm but gentle determination to maintain your attention and intention.

Wu Ji Posture

Proper body alignment provides the ways and means for smooth energetic flow. In Tai Ji and Qigong, this proper body alignment is called the Wu Ji Posture, where "wu" means none, and "ji" (the same "ji" of Tai Ji or Tai Chi) means extreme. Hence this is the way of standing that has no extremes. It is sometimes called the "emptiness" posture. It is commonly used for beginning and ending movements, and it can also be used alone, as a standing meditation. Here are the steps to achieving the Wu Ji Posture:

1. Stand with your feet approximately shoulders-width apart; toes pointing straight ahead.

2. Allow your knees to relax; do not lock them.

3. Roll the tip of the sacrum under as if sitting down. This subtle movement lengthens the spine and opens the Gate of Life point (Ming Men, located on the spine opposite the navel).

4. Drop the shoulders and allow them to spread, like wings, widening the back.

5. Tuck in the chin, and imagine the top of your head (the Crown Point) being pulled upward.

6. Feel your weight pressing down through the balls of the feet to stimulate the kidney meridian.

7. Breathe slowly, smoothly, evenly, and deeply, inhaling and exhaling like a balloon through your lower abdominal region.

8. Empty your mind.

9. Place the tip of the tongue on the roof of the mouth behind the teeth, as if saying "N."

As mind, breath, and body become calm and centered through these three regulations, notice yourself becoming more alert. This is the flow of Qi.

Pulling Down the Heavens

The practice of "pulling down the heavens" is a staple of Qigong practice. I recommend doing it before and after every practice. It is a simple, sweeping movement.

1. Starting from the Wu Ji posture, as you inhale, raise or float your arms wide to the side, palms up, gently curved.

2. At the top of your reach, as you begin to exhale, turn your palms over and bring the arms down, palms passing in front of your abdomen.

3. Do this three times, in a continuous sweeping motion. On the first sweep, you might picture pure white light flowing down the outside of your body; on the second sweep, imagine pure white light flowing through the inside of your body; and on the third sweep, imagine pure white light flowing both inside and outside—suffusing your entire body.

4. End the sequence by returning to the Wu Ji posture.

White Pearl Meditation

This meditation will help ground your energy as well as restore your vitality; it specifically enhances Kidney Essence, which will be discussed in Chapter 10. It is good to do anytime you feel depleted. It is also a good basic daily practice. The White Pearl Meditation is also available on CD or on iTunes.

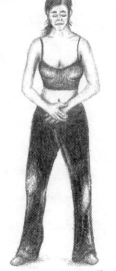

1. Assume the Wu Ji posture; remember the Three Regulations. Check your alignment, head to toe, and look for any tension. Relax down the body, front, back, and center.

2. Pull Down the Heavens three times.

3. Breathe through the nose into the lower Dan Tian, located about one inch below the navel. Keep your breath long, smooth, even, and deep. Allow and feel the breath simultaneously expanding the abdomen to the front, back, left, and right. This expansion and contraction will fill the lower Dan Tian with both breath and Qi.

4. Imagine your lower Dan Tian as a white luminescent pearl of incredible beauty. As you breathe, the energy from the heavens and your tissues fills the lower Dan Tian. See and feel this pearl becoming brighter and denser with each inhalation and exhalation.

5. Now use this energy to restore the "battery" of your own energy system, the kidneys. As you inhale, see and feel the pearl expand with pure, luminous white light. As you exhale, see and feel the energy from the pearl fill and restore the left and right kidneys.

6. Continue this breathing pattern for 10–15 minutes.

7. To finish, Pull Down the Heavens three times.

Notes

1. In step 5, you may place your hands on your abdomen. You might feel warmth all around your waist, as this corresponds to the Belt Vessel (an Extraordinary Meridian).

2. The most common error people make in doing this exercise is not pulling the breath down deeply enough. If you don't pull it down into the abdomen—that is, if you breathe only into the chest—you may experience gas and discomfort in your stomach.

3. In breathing, feel your lower abdomen (one inch below the navel,

roughly corresponding to the Lower Dan Tian) expand in all directions—front, back, right side, left side. This means it is totally relaxed. (Actually, it is good to breathe like this all day long.)

4. While best done in the Wu Ji standing posture, the Pearl Meditation can also be done sitting or lying down. For sitting, be sure to press up the Crown Point of the head; in both cases, remember to touch the tip of the tongue to the upper palate of your mouth behind the teeth. If you are tired it is better to sit and do the meditation than not to do it at all.

5. This is a good general practice, beneficial after any other daily routine or meditation.

GENERAL COMMENT

No matter how simple a practice may seem, it can have a profound effect. Just because you do not feel anything, do not think nothing is happening, especially in the early stages when you may not be very sensitive. Maintain your grounding, proper posture, sincere intention and focused attention. With patience and perseverance you will certainly make progress.

Chapter 2: THE NATURE OF QI

In Chinese metaphysics, Qi is the subtle energy that creates, sustains, activates and animates the universe. It is said to be present in inanimate objects, like rocks, as well as in living things like plants and animals, as well as in the subtle states of immaterial things like the air, light, sound and thought. It is said to have different qualities or to be of different types; some of these are positive and nurturing for living beings, others are negative.

In our bodies, our overall Qi can be subdivided in different ways. At conception there are four influences: Heavenly Qi, which is the basis of human consciousness; the natural vitality of the sperm and egg of the parents; and the energy of the time, place and environment. This is somewhat comparable to the Western concept of genetics.

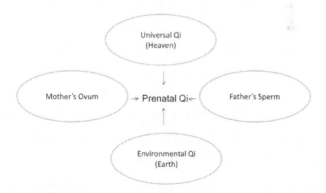

Prenatal Qi is the general name for the energy you were born with and is expressed in the Kidney Qi. In other words, in Chinese medicine your constitution is expressed in the energy of your Kidney, which we will discuss later. If your parents and ancestors were healthy, then you are likely to be healthy. After birth, you are nourished by what the Chinese call Postnatal Qi, which is derived from the Qi of the food you eat and the Qi of the air you breathe. All of these energies are part of our overall Qi. The quality of each individual component contributes to the overall state of your health.

Essentially, if the Qi is strong, flowing and coherent, life flourishes. In the Chinese understanding, a person basically lives on two sources of energy: Prenatal Qi, the amount and quality of which was fixed at conception, and Postnatal Qi, which is under your control. The more you can conserve your Prenatal Qi, the longer you live and the better the quality of your life. The better your Postnatal Qi is, the less you use up of your Prenatal Qi. In other words, if you eat well, breathe clean air, live in a good place, you will thrive on Postnatal Qi. But if you eat fast food, live erratically, indulge in anger and anxiety, without enough Postnatal Qi, your body will use Prenatal Qi instead, ultimately degrading and shortening your life. Whenever your Qi becomes stagnant, deficient or scatters, this opens the door for disease and, ultimately, for death.

The purpose of Qigong practice is to harmonize and nurture our Qi. The first step is learning to feel Qi. First, we become aware of what is happening in our bodies—especially in individual organ systems. This awareness does not come overnight; developing it is a lifelong practice. But even at the beginning, you should get a flash of it, a sense of the possibilities. Then, through meditations and exercises, with steady determination and regular practice, you can nurture that flash of light into a beacon. Once you are aware, you can take the second step, which is to act appropriately. This course will give you exercises to develop your sensitivity to Qi, and also methods to balance the disharmonies that you encounter.

Interestingly, as you become more aware of what is happening in your own body, you will become more sensitive to the Qi around you, in the environment, for example, and in other beings—people, animals, plants. As your sensitive self grows, your intuitive and psychic selves grow as well. You then have the chance to improve your health on all levels. All Qi is connected.

BODY AWAKENING EXERCISES

The following three Body Awakening Exercises are another foundation of my Qigong practice. I recommend doing these before any Qigong session to help bring body and mind together, in a centered state and to help loosen the body to allow the free flow of Qi. It will make all your subsequent practices more effective.

1. Begin by assuming the Wu Ji posture, and remembering the Three Regulations.

2. Pull Down the Heavens three times.

Tossing a Stone

1. From Wu Ji posture, lift your arms out to the side until they are shoulder height, palms down ("T" position). Inhale.

2. As you exhale, turn your upper torso to one side and swing the opposite arm, palm up, as though tossing a stone, while the other arm swings behind you.

3. Inhale as you return to the "T" position.

4. As you exhale, repeat on the other side. In other words, if you turn to the right, your left arm will swing in front and to the right as though tossing a stone, while your right arm will swing behind you.

5. Repeat in a continuous rhythm, synchronized with your breathing, first one side then the other. Do this 3-9 times on each side.

6. End by Pulling Down the Heavens three times.

The Heel Drop

7. From Wu Ji posture, begin lightly bouncing on the balls of your feet.

8. As you bounce, mentally visit each major joint of your body and

release any tension there. Picture the tension descending down and out of the body. Start with your ankles, then move up to knees, then hips, and end at the heart center. Then go to fingers, and travel up the arms, through wrists, elbows, and shoulders, ending at the neck.

9. Stop bouncing. Imagine gold light rising through your body.

10. Rise up on the balls of your feet, inhale, pulling the light up to and beyond the top of your head. Then, suddenly, sharply drop on your heels, releasing all tension into the earth.

11. Repeat this 3-9 times.

12. End by Pulling Down the Heavens three times.

Shaking the Tree

13. From the Wu Ji posture, raise your arms out in front of you, parallel, about shoulder height.

14. With hands in loose fists, pull your hands alternately to your chest, as though hauling in something at the end of a rope.

15. Repeat, continuously, starting with slow large movements, each successive one faster and smaller until your hands are at your chest.

16. Immediately shake your whole body, head to toe. The more relaxed you are the more you will feel the vibration throughout your whole body, including your internal organs.

17. Repeat 3-9 times.

18. End by Pulling Down the Heavens three times.

CENTER AND BALANCE MEDITATION

The Center and Balance Meditation is the basic exercise for developing a relationship with your own body as well as with the cosmic energies of Heaven and Earth. It asks you to be present in the now, in your body and not in your head. It has four stages. The Center and Balance Meditation is also available on CD or on iTunes.

1. Start with the Three Regulations: Steady breath, relaxed mind, Wu Ji posture (feet shoulder width, shoulders relaxed, tailbone tucked, Crown Point rising).

2. Focus your attention on the front of your forehead in between the eyebrows. Imagine warm oil melting down the front of your body covering everything in its path. Feel this oil absorbing impurities, leaving your cells clean and vibrant. Once the oil reaches your feet feel it run off and down deep into the ground.

3. Now focus on the back of your head. Imagine smooth, warm oil flowing down the whole backside of your body. Feel as much in the back as you did in the front. Feel this warm oil cover and cleanse every cell and tissue of your body, again flowing off your feet, then deep into the earth.

4. Next focus attention on the top of the head, what is called the Crown Point (GV20) in Chinese medicine. Connect with your higher power. Imagine a white light from heaven entering through the Crown Point and flowing down through the body, cleansing all the internal organs. Imagine the white light permeating every tissue inside your body. Imagine it going through your head, down your spine, through your abdomen, down your legs and deep into the ground.

5. Imagine that your feet melt into the earth, leaving you standing in a sea of liquid energy about the height of your ankles.

6. Imagine roots growing from the centers of bottoms of your feet, what are called the Bubbling Well points in Chinese medicine

(K1). These roots connect deep into the earth, twice the height of the body. This will give you a strong connection with both Heaven and Earth.

7. Inhale, imagining energy from the earth going up the roots, up through your legs, expanding into your Lower Dan Tian. Then, exhale and imagine the energy going back down into the ground. Repeat this over and over, filling up the entire lower abdomen, then releasing the energy down into the earth.

8. End by spreading both arms to the side, raising them up over your head, and then bringing them down in front, finally resting your palms on top of each other on your lower abdomen.

Chapter 3: THE MERIDIAN SYSTEM

The word meridian, as used in Chinese Medicine, entered the English language as a French translation of the Chinese medical term jing-luo. "Jing" means to go through or a thread in a fabric; "luo" means something that connects or attaches or a net.

Meridians are the channels or pathways that carry Qi throughout the body. They are different from physical blood vessels; instead they are an invisible network of subtle energy pathways. In Chinese meridian theory, these channels represent a kind of informational network. Qi moves along them, connecting all of the organs, as well as the interior and exterior of the body. The amount and quality of flow of energy along these pathways determines the health of the body; deficiency, excess, stagnation and blockage are the typical problems. The various therapies of Chinese medicine address these problems at specific points, based on the details of the meridian system.

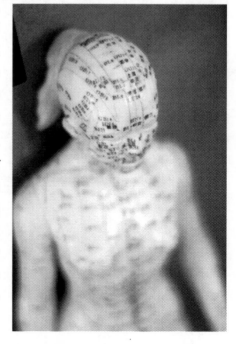

The meridian system of Chinese medical theory comprises twelve Regular Meridians and eight Extraordinary Meridians. The Extraordinary Meridians, or Vessels, are actually part of the regular Meridians, and will be covered later.

The regular meridians are named according to the major organs of the body. Each meridian is a channel of energy associated with a particular organ; the energy runs between points where the flow can be influenced.

The Regular Meridians are found to function in pairs, one Yin and one Yang. The meaning of Yin and Yang will be explained in the next chapter; for now, simply think of these Yin and Yang components as being closely related, like brother and sister. The Yin meridians are located on the inner aspects of the body; in them, Qi flows upward. The Yang meridians are located on the outer aspects of the body; in them, Qi flows downward. Each pair corresponds to one of the Five Elements, another set of concepts that will be explained later (Chapter 6). The main point to understand for now is that Qi flows through the body in particular pathways, described in English as meridians. These meridians function in pairs, and each pair is associated with certain qualities and characteristics that are true both in the body and in nature.

The Twelve Meridians in Pairs according to the Five Elements:						
Element	**FIRE**	**EARTH**	**METAL**	**WATER**	**WOOD**	**(Extra)**
YIN	Heart	Spleen	Lungs	Kidney	Liver	Pericardium*
YANG	Small Intestine	Stomach	Large Intestine	Urinary Bladder	Gall Bladder	Triple Burner*

*The Pericardium is the tissue surrounding the heart, while the Triple Burner is a conceptual organ unique to the Chinese medical system. These will be described in a later chapter.

BRUSHING THE MERIDIANS

In this practice we will use our hands to trace the meridians. This should harmonize and stimulate the flow of Qi. We will move upward along the Yin Meridians (insides of the body and limbs) as we inhale, and we will move our hands downward along the Yang Meridians (outsides of the body and limbs), exhaling. Use a flat hand, palm facing the body. You may actually touch the body, or you may keep the hand just above the surface of the body. Clothes don't matter. Move at a speed consistent with your breath.

Preliminary

1. Start with the Three Regulations: Steady breath, relaxed mind, Wu Ji posture (feet shoulder width, shoulders relaxed, tailbone tucked, Crown Point rising).

2. Pull Down the Heavens three times. You may lightly bounce to relax and loosen the body.

Upper body

3. Begin with arms out to the side in a "T" position.

4. As you inhale, bring hands together in front of the body, and draw the hands up the opposite arm. That is, the right hand moves up the outside of the left arm while the left hand moves up the outside of the right arm.

5. At the shoulder, continue moving the hands up the sides of the head (arms will be crossed).

6. At the top of the head, the hands uncross.

7. Exhale as you let your hands flow naturally down the front of the body, then down the outsides of the legs.

8. Roll up on the balls of your feet as you flick your hands outward and say "SHUU" releasing your breath with a sharp exhalation. Imagine that you are throwing any bad energy you have collected on your hands into the earth.

Lower body

9. Now lean over, and put your hands on your ankles, left hand on left instep and right hand on right instep. As you inhale, move your hands up the inside of your legs to the groin.

10. Cross your hands, then move up into the armpits.

11. Exhale. As you do so, draw each hand down the opposite arm, down the inside of the forearms, until you pull your hands apart, palms facing each other.

12. Repeat from Step 1.

13. To end the practice, Pull Down the Heavens three times.

NOTES

1. Chinese texts recommend repeating this exercise 9-36 times (i.e., multiples of 9, which is a harmonic number).

2. You can perform the same practice using cupped hands and slapping the body, rather than brushing. In this case, slap the body firmly, with conviction, to stimulate the flow of energy.

3. You can do this on other people, either brushing or tapping. Either way, it should be an enjoyable and invigorating experience.

4. This is a good practice for anyone when they are physically "tight" or tense because it will stimulate the nerves and improve blood circulation.

5. This is also a good practice to do when you feel a cold or flu coming on, or when you sense any other imbalance in your energy. It should restore harmony quickly.

Feeling bad can be good

Do not expect always to feel good immediately after doing Qigong. By harmonizing energy flow you are forcing issues to resolve themselves. Sometimes this can be uncomfortable. The practice is safe; continue, but perhaps more gently or more slowly. Eventually you should feel much better than before. You will not always know why—and knowing why doesn't seem to matter—but, in the long run, in my experience, you will definitely feel better.

Chapter 4: YIN AND YANG OF THE ORGANS

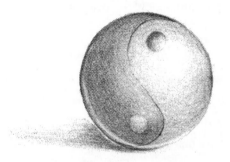

Yin and Yang are philosophical concepts based on relativity. While they are fundamental to Chinese philosophy, they are foreign to Western philosophical thought. Generally speaking, Western philosophy seeks absolutes. It seeks to determine what is true and what is not true. In contrast Chinese philosophy is interested in relative relationships, and these relationships are described as Yin and Yang. Just as something is big or small according to what you compare it to; similarly something is Yin or Yang according to what you compare it to.

It is said that Yin and Yang were first defined as the two sides of a hill, one dark, the other light; one cool, the other hot. This led to the observation that every phenomenon is constantly cycling between two opposite poles. Night becomes day, which becomes night. Heaven is yang, round; Earth is yin, square. More active, brighter, more expansive is relatively more Yang than that which is quiet, dark, contracting. Yin and Yang are at the same time opposites and complements. Further, Yin contains the root of Yang and Yang contains the root of Yin; Yin at its extreme becomes Yang, while

Yang at its extreme becomes Yin. For example, frantic activity (Yang) often leads to collapse (Yin). Yin and Yang are interdependent by definition, and they are constantly interchanging, one into the other.

In the human body, the early Chinese doctors found that the meridians functioned in pairs, one being relatively Yin and the other relatively Yang. Thus, the Stomach and Spleen worked together, with the Stomach being more active/Yang while the Spleen was relatively Yin. The Large Intestines and Lungs worked together, Small Intestines and Heart, Gall Bladder and Liver, and Urinary Bladder and Kidneys—all being Yang and Yin organs, respectively.

The Chinese classics view the Yin organs as more precious than the Yang. While Yang is responsible for heat and is the motive force which creates change and transformation, it is the nurturing nature of Yin that supports life. It is the nature of Yang to go to excess; it is the nature of Yang to be bold, to demand attention. In contrast, it is the nature of Yin to become deficient, to withdraw, to fail without fanfare. Supplying deficient Yin is generally more difficult than curbing excess Yang. Thus, much of Chinese medicine—and Qigong exercises—particularly target those precious Yin organs and their energy.

MASSAGING THE YANG ORGANS

This exercise massages all the Yang organs—which is essentially the entire digestive system. Thus it is great for all digestive discomforts or complaints, both acute, such as nausea, as well as chronic problems such as constipation and heartburn.

1. Begin by standing in the Wu Ji posture, feet shoulder distance apart, tail bone tucked, chin tucked so as to raise the crown of the head, relaxed and balanced.

2. Raise your arms in front of you to shoulder level while you inhale through the nose into the lower abdomen. Keep the abdomen relaxed, and allow it to expand as if fills with air.

3. When ready to exhale, contract the abdomen, expelling the air as your arms swing back using about 70% power (that is, let inertia help carry them back).

4. Allow the arms to swing back up in front to repeat the exercise.

5. Repeat 50 times at first, gradually increasing to 150 times.

NOTES

1. Breathing should be natural, such that the swinging is also in a natural, easy rhythm.

2. For acute problems, do this exercise as needed. For chronic issues, do it once per day, ideally in the morning.

3. You can also do this exercise from a seated position (although standing is preferred).

CASE HISTORY

A woman in her late 50s came in, very upset because of pressure in her abdomen diagnosed by her physician as a prolapsed (fallen) uterus. Her doctor advised a hysterectomy. She also had fibroids, was prone to yeast infections and reported she bruised easily. I assessed the fundamental problem as deficiency disrupting the Spleen. I recommended she radically change her diet, eliminating all cold, raw foods and all pasta, breads, sugars (including fruit). I did Medical Qigong to help warm and raise the uterus. After three sessions the uterus had returned to its normal position. And she has never returned to her previous diet.

Chapter 5: THE VESSELS AND GATES

There are eight Extraordinary Meridians that help regulate the flow of energy through the body. They do this in two ways. First, they connect the main meridians. Their connections ensure that energy flows smoothly throughout the body, and facilitate communication between the organs, supporting their proper function. Second, the Extraordinary Meridians serve as reservoirs of energy, which means they can supply deficiencies or absorb excesses in the main meridians. Because of this function, they are also called vessels. Two of the most important Extraordinary Meridians are the **Governing Vessel** and the **Conception Vessel**. The Governing Vessel runs up the back of the body, from the perineum to the cleft above the teeth, while the Conception Vessel runs up the front of the body from the perineum to the depression beneath the protrusion of the lower lip (The perineum is the anatomical point between the sex glands and the anal sphincter). Thus, together, these two meridians encircle the body on its vertical axis. Both run very close to the surface of the body. The path of these meridians also coincides with the network of the central nervous system (CNS). Stimulating the CNS will fill the vessels, and by extension all the meridians the vessels supply.

Along these vessels, there are certain specific points where Qi—as well as blood, other body fluids, and emotions—tend to get blocked. These points are known as gates. There are seven gates of particular importance in Qigong practice:

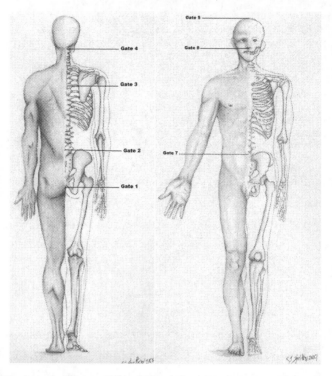

1ˢᵗ Gate: Perineum (Conception Vessel 1, or CV1) located between the sex glands and the anal sphincter muscle.

2ⁿᵈ Gate: Gate of Life or Mingmen (Governing Vessel 4, or GV4) located on the spine, exactly opposite to the navel.

3ʳᵈ Gate: Shendao (Governing Vessel 11, or GV11) located between the shoulder blades.

4ᵗʰ Gate: Fengfu (Governing Vessel 16, or GV16) located at the base of the skull.

5ᵗʰ Gate: Crown Point or Baihui (Governing Vessel 20, or GV20) located at the top of the head.

6ᵗʰ Gate: Mouth Point or Yinjiao (Governing Vessel 28, or GV28) located at the junction of the upper lip and the gum.

7ᵗʰ Gate: Sea of Qi or Qi Hai (Conception Vessel 6) located about an inch and a half below the navel.

A third important Extraordinary Meridian is the **Belt Vessel,** which encircles the body at the waist.

Stimulating and regulating the flow of energy in the vessels helps regulate flow of energy throughout the body in all the regular meridians. The meditation known as the Micro-Cosmic Orbit, or the Jupiter Cycle Meditation or Small Heaven Breathing, specifically activates the Governing and Conception Vessels.

MICRO-COSMIC ORBIT MEDITATION

The purpose of this meditation is to facilitate and reinforce the flow of Qi in the Conception and Governing Vessels. The first step is simply to become aware of the movement of the Qi; in later stages, you can develop power in guiding Qi. Ancient sages said that, with sincere practice, it will take one hundred days to fully open these two channels or meridians. The time it takes is not important; even one day of practice will bring benefit!

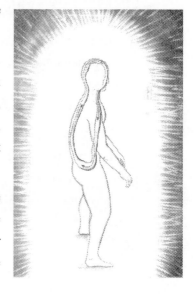

1. Start with the Three Regulations: Steady breath, relaxed mind, Wu Ji posture (feet shoulder width, shoulders relaxed and broad, tailbone tucked, Crown Point rising).

2. Place the tongue place on the roof of the mouth behind the teeth. Squeeze the anal sphincter muscle, and otherwise relax the body.

3. As you inhale, guide the Qi up the spine (i.e., up the Governing Vessel), to the crown of the head. If you cannot feel the Qi, imagine it. You may imagine it as light or a color or as blood or fluids moving upward.

4. As you exhale, guide the Qi from the Crown Point down the front of the face, entering the upper palate of the mouth to the point where the tongue touches the palate.

5. Continuing to exhale, guide the Qi down the front of the body (i.e., the Conception Vessel) to the perineum.

6. When the Qi reaches the perineum, repeat the exercise—that is, inhale bringing the Qi up the spine, then exhale bringing it over the crown of the head to the tongue tip, and down the front to the perineum.

7. Repeat the exercise continuously. At the end, with your mind, bring the Qi to the lower Dan Tian and store it there.

NOTES

1. Initially, practice this meditation for 10-15 minutes per day.

2. At the beginning, when you may not feel the flow of Qi, use the length of one inhalation to visualize bringing the Qi from the base of the spine to the crown of the head. Later, you can do it much faster, especially when you are aware of the Qi and its natural tendencies.

3. You may practice the Micro-cosmic Orbit in any position (standing, sitting, or lying down), and at any time. For example, you might do it any time you are waiting, as when stopped at a traffic light or standing in line at a store or even while watching TV.

My personal experience

Although the ancient texts say it should take one hundred days (about three months) to open the Gates and feel the flow of Qi, for me it took six months. I did the meditation regularly, every day, and felt nothing... until one day I felt the tip of my tongue pulsating or vibrating where it rested on the roof of my mouth. Since then I have gradually been able to increase my awareness. First, I could feel the Qi throughout its route in the Governing and Conception Vessels, then I could feel it in other organs. I believe doing the Micro-cosmic Orbit is a fundamental first step in following, and eventually, controlling one's Qi.

Chapter 6: FIVE ELEMENTS IN DETAIL

The Chinese theory of the Five Elements arises from the observation of ancient sages that all phenomena in the universe are the products of movement of the five qualities of Fire, Earth, Metal, Water, and Wood. From the original void of Wu Ji, arose Yin-Yang. Yin-Yang within this Wu Ji generates the Three Treasures: Heaven, Earth, and Man. The energy continues to unfold to the four divisions of Yin and Yang. These four divisions plus the Earth Element give us five phases of energy, commonly known as the Five Elements. From the Five Elements come the "ten thousand things" or our material world. In Chinese medicine, Five Element theory has had considerable influence on physiology, pathology, diagnosis, treatment and pharmacology. It has also been applied in the realms of Feng Shui and astrology.

Each of the Five Elements has specific characteristics and associations, as observed in nature over two millennia. Throughout this book I will capitalize these five words when they refer to the Chinese concepts and not to physical objects. Thus:

> **Fire** has the traits of flaming upward, expansion, heat, dispersion and dissipation.

> **Earth** is the sowing, reaping and bringing forth of all phenomena; it carries the traits of harmonizing and balance; it is essentially neutral.

> **Metal** is the working of change; it has the qualities of purification, refinement, elimination, reform, and gravity.

> **Water** has the traits of contraction, collection, condensation.

> **Wood** has the characteristics of growth, initiation, release, and rejuvenation.

The Five Elements relate to each other in three cycles: the creative cycle, the controlling cycle, and the destructive cycle, as depicted in Figures 10-12. Understanding these natural patterns of metamorphosis can help explain how organ systems affect one another, and how to treat one system through a related system. They also help us understand how problems with one organ system can affect others. Meridian theory, together with Five Element theory, are how the Chinese describe and explain the interactions of the human body as a dynamic, holistic system.

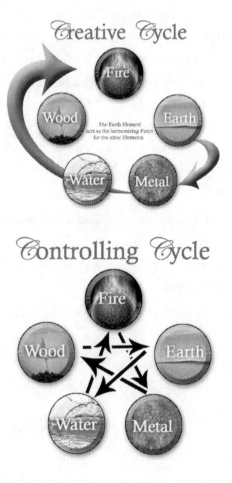

Destructive Cycle

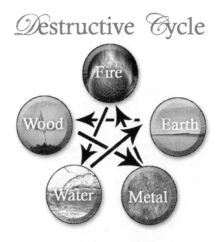

COLLECTING HEAVEN AND EARTH

The purpose of this exercise is to absorb heavenly Yang and earthly Yin energy, and then bring them together in harmony. It is the opening exercise for the five Organ Cleansing Exercises which we will do next.

1. Start with the Three Regulations: Steady breath, relaxed mind, Wu Ji posture (feet shoulder width, shoulders relaxed and broad, tailbone tucked, Crown Point rising).

2. Spread the arms wide at shoulder level, in a "T" position, with palms facing up.

3. Raise the arms up over the head, palms facing each other.

4. As if rounding over a big ball, bend forward from the hips, keeping shoulders relaxed and keeping the chin tucked toward the chest. Let the arms follow the movement.

5. When you have bent forward as far as you can, slowly drop the arms and hands toward the ground; let them dangle. Do not lock the knees, let them be loose.

6. Bend the knees as you curl up to a standing position, one vertebra at a time.

7. Repeat the exercise 36 times.

CASE HISTORY

I sometimes volunteer at elementary schools to teach kids about the different forms of Qigong and Tai Chi. A few weeks later the teacher called to report what had happened on a museum field trip. On the way, the kids were getting quite rowdy and out of control, until one of the class leaders suggested, "Hey! Let's do that practice of Collecting Heaven and Earth that Mr. Shelton taught us!" So the whole class started doing this exercise in the middle of downtown San Jose. As if by magic, the teacher reported, all the kids calmed down and the rest of the trip went smoothly.

Chapter 7: FIRE ELEMENT

Yin Organs:	**Heart**	**Hours: 11 am- 1 pm**
	Pericardium	**Hours: 7-9 pm**
Yang Organs:	**Small Intestine**	**Hours: 1-3 pm**
	Triple Burner	**Hours: 9-11 pm**

Starting with this Chapter, I will be discussing each of the Five Elements in terms of the meridians and organ systems with which they are associated. Because the Yin organs are considered the most precious (for reasons mentioned in Chapter 5), for each Element I will focus on its associated Yin organ. I will follow the creative cycle (as shown in Fig. 10), starting with the Fire Element.

Finally, one more important note for all the chapters that follow: The Chinese references are not exactly the same as the Western labels for the anatomical organs. For example, when the TCM (traditional Chinese medicine) refers to the Kidney, it is referring to the energy of the Kidney system—not necessarily to the physical organ, the kidney. Thus, if a Chinese doctor tells a patient that he/she has Kidney problems he does not necessarily mean she has kidney disease. To remind the reader of this distinction, I will capitalize the organ names when they refer to the Chinese concept, and not capitalize them when they refer to the physical organ.

The Fire Element has two pairs of meridians associated with it. One pair is the Heart and Small Intestine; the other pair is the Pericardium (anatomically, the pericardium is the tissue surrounding the heart) and the Triple Burner. The Triple Burner is a conceptual energy system unique to Chinese medical theory. It has hours of activity, specific functions, points of access and control, etc., exactly like the other meridians, but it has no physical form.

In Chinese medicine, the **Heart** is said to rule the blood and blood vessels. While the Liver is said to be the Controller of blood, the Heart is said to be the Governor. This means that the Liver allows blood to move, while the Heart determines where the blood needs to go. The **Pericardium** refers to the protective tissue of the heart. External pathogenic factors as well as emotions mostly attack the pericardium before they affect the heart.

The heart organ is located in the chest to the left. It is believed in TCM that the Heart energy is particularly important among all the organs, as it controls the other viscera and bowels. The Heart has Yin and Yang aspects. The Yin refers to the blood controlled by the heart. The Yang refers to the actual function, the heat, and Qi of the heart. The main functions of the Heart are controlling blood circulation, taking charge of mental activities, and producing sweat as the fluid of the heart. In terms of other body parts, the condition of the Heart is particularly expressed in the tongue and face.

- Controlling blood circulation

Blood vessels are the tubes in which blood flows. They are linked to the heart, creating a closed system. TCM says that it is the Qi of the heart that keeps it beating and sending blood through blood vessels. When the Qi is sufficient, the heart can keep a normal rate and strength. The pulse of the heart reflects much about the Qi of the body and of the condition of the internal organs. Indeed, pulse diagnosis is an important form of assessment in TCM. You can think of assessing the pulse like assessing the flow of water in a hose. The condition of the hose—is it flexible or stiff? Fully open or clogged?—as well as the power of the pump—does it pump evenly or irregularly, is it strong or weak? Etc.—will determine the quality and nature of the flow of water inside. A weak and empty pulse shows deficiency of the Qi of the heart. A fine and weak pulse shows deficiency of the blood of the heart. A rough and rhythmical pulse shows decline of the blood of the heart.

- Taking charge of mental activities

The Fire Element rules the firing of the brain's neurons, the synapses, and the receptor sites. TCM asserts that nervous activities like thinking depend on the function of the heart. When the functions of the heart are normal, the person will have a healthy consciousness and healthy mental activities. Abnormalities, like insanity, may be brought on by insufficiency of blood. Treatment for such kinds of mental problems is determined through analysis of the Heart condition.

- Sweat as the fluid of the Heart

Body fluid is the fundamental component of blood and sweat. TCM says that profuse sweating means the heart is using a lot of blood and Qi, which may result in palpitations and violent beatings of the heart. Too much sweating depletes Yin and injures Yang of the heart. , Those who have a lack of Yin in the heart are likely to sweat at night. At the same time, sweating does not always indicate heart problems. In TCM no condition can be diagnosed from just one symptom.

- Relationship with the tongue and face

TCM believes that the condition of the Heart is expressed on the tongue and in the complexion of the face. With its many blood vessels, the face readily shows the condition of the heart. A rosy face, pink tongue, and sparkling eyes show that the heart is functioning well and the person's spirit is strong. A white face and pale tongue suggest the heart is not functioning well. Stagnation of the Heart energy can be represented in a face that is blue and a dark purple tongue.

On the psychological level, the Heart is also responsible for a person's appropriate interactions in time and place. It allows for manners and propriety. On the emotional level, Heart energy that is in balance is expressed as the positive virtues of love and compassion; out of balance, it is expressed as over-excitation and frantic activity.

FIRE ELEMENT IMBALANCE

>>Physical signs:

- ☯ Lackluster eyes
- ☯ Heart palpitations
- ☯ Mental illness (bipolar, manic)
- ☯ Low or high blood pressure
- ☯ Dizziness

>>Emotional signs:

- ☯ Anxiety with situations and people
- ☯ Forgetfulness
- ☯ Shyness
- ☯ Sense of vulnerability
- ☯ Jumpiness or chattiness
- ☯ Hysteria

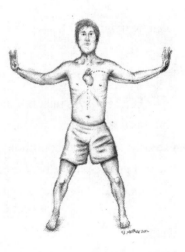

PATH OF THE HEART MERIDIAN

The Heart meridian has three branches, each of which begins in the heart. Two of the branches are internal; one runs through the diaphragm to connect to the small intestine, while a second branch runs upward along the side of the throat to the eye. The third, external branch runs across the chest from the heart to the lung, then descends and emerges in the underarm. Thus, on the surface of the body, it begins at the front crease of the armpit, runs down the inside of the arm, across the wrist and palm, and terminates at the inside tip of the little finger where it connects with the Small Intestine meridian.

USEFUL ACUPOINT ON THE HEART MERIDIAN

HT 9: This point is located at the tip of the pinky finger, on the inner edge of the fingernail. Holding or massaging this point will normalize heart rate. Thus, whenever you feel your heart rate rise—for physical causes, such as a vigorous workout, or for emotional causes, such as stage fright—hold your pinky and breathe deeply. You may also say the Heart sound, "HAAA", for extra help in restoring normal heart rate.

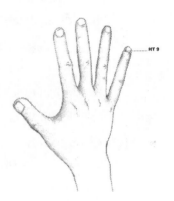

HEART CLEANSING EXERCISE

This exercise particularly clears and harmonizes the energy of the Heart. It is useful for addressing any of the physical and emotional complaints listed above. You may use it for chronic conditions or acute situations, or you may use it simply to keep your Heart energy flowing smoothly.

THE MOVEMENT:

1. Start with the Three Regulations: Steady breath, relaxed mind, Wu Ji posture (feet shoulder width, shoulders relaxed and broad,

tailbone tucked, Crown Point rising). The tongue should be lightly touching the roof of the mouth behind the upper teeth.

2. Pull Down the Heavens three times.

3. Place the hands comfortably in front of the body, as though cradling a baby, at the height of the lower abdomen. The right hand should be on top, fingers touching palms, facing upward.

4. Turn your upper torso to the left. As you turn your left arm rises, the forearm rotates to point the palm outward while, at the same time, the right arm pushes to the left, under the left arm, palm facing outward. (For those who do martial arts, this is a classic "block and punch" type of move.)

5. When you've reached a comfortable extension, allow the arms to come back, returning to the starting position, but this time with the left hand on top, palm pointing down toward the right palm pointing up.

6. Now mirror Step 3 on the right side. That is, turn your torso to the right. As you turn, raise your right arm, rotating the palm outward as the left arm pushes under it to the right, palm facing outward.

7. Return to center, and repeat, left and right, at an even gentle pace, 3-36 times.

8. Close by Pulling Down the Heavens three times.

NOTES

1. To increase the efficacy of the exercise, you may say the Heart sound, "HAAA" while exhaling.

2. Breathing is a key aspect here; be sure to inhale as you come to center, exhale as you turn and push out.

CASE HISTORY

A middle-aged man who had had several heart attacks was working out at the gym. Because of his previous history, he was required to wear a heart monitor. During one session his heart rate shot up to 180 beats per minute. His trainer grabbed the man's pinky fingers and squeezed. Within a minute, the man's heart rate had returned to a more normal level of 80.

Chapter 8: EARTH ELEMENT

Yin Organ:	**Spleen**	**Hours: 9-11 am**
Yang Organ:	**Stomach**	**Hours: 7-9 am**

The Spleen in Chinese medicine is different from the anatomical organ as described in Western medicine. TCM says that the Spleen is located in the middle of the body cavity and is the main organ of digestion. Its Yin aspect is its material structure while its Yang aspect is its function. The Spleen's function, which is absolutely fundamental to the health of the body, is transforming food and liquid into blood. The Spleen is also responsible for containing organs in their proper places, such as the blood in its vessels and uterus and anus in their positions. The Spleen has relationships with the muscles, limbs, and lips.

- Transporting, distributing, and transforming nutrients

TCM states that, after going through the stomach, food enters the Spleen where it is separated into what is useful and what is not. The waste travels through the pylorus to the small intestine. What is not waste is said to "rise" to the Lungs where it is combined with air and sent to the Heart to produce blood. If the Spleen is not functioning properly, a person may suffer from lack of appetite, indigestion, fullness and distension in the epigastrium (upper middle section of the abdomen), loose stools, lassitude, and/or loss of weight, among other symptoms. The Spleen also absorbs and transports water. If the Spleen cannot absorb water properly, the body retains water, resulting in edema, dampness, and/or diarrhea. Thus the Spleen absorbs both food and water at the same time, and both functions are connected. An abnormal function of one will lead to an abnormal function of the other.

- Keeping blood circulating within the vessels

The Spleen keeps the blood circulating normally within the vessels. If there is lack of Qi, the blood will not flow normally and will escape from the vessels. When this happens, it can result in such symptoms as blood in the stool, uterine bleeding, or spontaneous nosebleeds.

On a broader, energetic level, the Earth Element transforms food into the textures and activities of human life, and it is responsible for creative change in life. The Spleen in particular acts as the harmonizing force between all other organs. The Earth Element is associated with being centered in thought and action. Spleen energy which is in balance is expressed as the positive virtues of serenity, calmness, and centeredness. Out of balance, it is expressed as worry, over-intellectualizing and simply thinking too much. Conversely, anxiety and mental stress can cause problems in the Spleen and from there, the entire digestive system. Naturally sweet and bland foods nurture the Spleen.

EARTH ELEMENT IMBALANCE

>>Physical signs:

- Loose stools
- Anemia
- Major depressive disorders
- Allergies
- Underweight or overweight
- Diabetes

- Prolapse of any organ (e.g., uterus)
- Craving for sweet or starchy foods (carbohydrates)

>>Emotional signs:

- Apathy
- Brooding
- Over-intellectualizing or thinking
- Prolonged worry or anxiety

PATH OF THE SPLEEN MERIDIAN

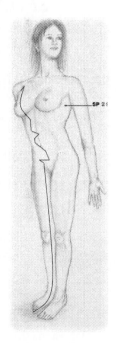

The Spleen meridian originates at the outside corner of the big toe. It then runs along the inside of the foot, turning in front of the inner anklebone. From there, it ascends straight up the lower leg behind the shinbone, up the inner aspect of the knee and thigh into the abdominal cavity. It runs internally to the spleen, and connects with the stomach. The main branch continues on the surface of the abdomen, running upward to the chest, where it again penetrates internally to follow the throat up to the root of the tongue, under which it spreads its Qi and blood. An internal branch leaves the stomach, passes upward through the diaphragm, and enters the heart, where it connects with the Heart meridian.

USEFUL ACUPOINTS ON THE SPLEEN MERIDIAN

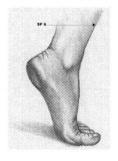

SP6: This point is located on the inside of the ankle, three fingers' width above the ankle bone. Massage this for digestive problems, particularly excess phlegm or mucus in the chest and also for arthritic pain, which

represents an accumulation of phlegm in the joints. Three Yin organ meridians converge at this point so it is particularly valuable for restoring balance in all Yin functions. This point can also be used to build or tonify blood.

SP21: This point is located under the armpit, more or less directly in the center. Massage this particularly for relieving the emotional aspects of Spleen imbalance, such as worry or brooding. This point connects directly with the Spleen, so is particularly potent.

SPLEEN CLEANSING EXERCISE

This exercise particularly clears and harmonizes the energy of the Spleen. On the physical level, it helps restore good digestive function. On the emotional level, it calms the mind. Practicing this movement can help reduce anxiety and worry, while re-establishing one's central stability. It is particularly recommended for people who spend a lot of time feeling worried or stressed or simply thinking too much.

THE MOVEMENT

1. Start with the Three Regulations: Steady breath, relaxed mind, Wu Ji posture (feet shoulder width, shoulders relaxed, tailbone tucked, Crown Point rising). The tongue should be lightly touching the roof of the mouth behind the upper teeth.

2. Pull Down the Heavens three times.

3. Bring the hands together in front of the body, just above the head, thumbs and index fingers together, forming the shape of a diamond.

4. Gaze upward through this diamond.

5. Continuing to gaze through the diamond, twist the torso to the left... back to center... then to the right. Repeat at a slow, deliberate, steady pace. Your hands should rotate around the center

of the diamond, and your knees should remain more or less facing forward. The main point is to compress and release your abdominal cavity, where the stomach and spleen are.

6. Repeat 3, 9 or 36 times.

7. Close by Pulling Down the Heavens three times.

NOTES

1. To increase the efficacy of the exercise, you may say the Spleen sound while gazing through the diamond. The Spleen sound is: "HUUU".

2. Remember to breathe deeply into your Dan Tian.

3. The easiest way to keep the diamond still is to find something on the ceiling, or above you, that falls in the center of the diamond. Then, as you twist, make sure that point of focus remains at the center of the diamond.

4. The most common error with this exercise is failing to keep the shoulders relaxed. Feel the weight of your shoulder blades, and allow them simply fall.

CASE HISTORY

Parents brought in their 5-year old son because he was having chronic nosebleeds. The doctors recommended cauterizing the blood vessels. After talking to the boy, I learned he was very anxious about the prospect of starting kindergarten. Stress depletes Spleen energy; sugar was no doubt also involved—another stress on the Spleen. I recommended a change of diet, eliminating sugars and processed foods. I taught him the Spleen Cleansing Movement and suggested that, whenever he felt anxious, he should say the Spleen sound. The treatment worked, and the problem was resolved.

Chapter 9: METAL ELEMENT

Yin Organ:	**Lung**	**Hours: 3-5 am**
Yang Organ:	**Large Intestine**	**Hours: 5-7 am**

The Metal Element relates to not only the respiratory system, but also the immune system (including the lymphatic system), the large intestine (colon), and the skin. The Metal Element is said to control Wei Qi, also called Defensive Qi. This particular type of Qi has a shielding affect and thus is often considered analogous to our immune system.

Anatomically, the lungs are made up of two lobes located in the chest. They connect to the larynx, bronchi, and trachea, opening to the external environment through the nose. In Chinese medicine, the Lung is divided into the Yin of the Lung (the material structure) and the Qi of the Lung (the functions of the lung); the term "Yang of the lung" is rarely used. The Yang organ paired with the Lung is the Large Intestine. The function of both is particularly expressed in the quality of the skin and strength of the voice.

The Lungs are particularly involved with regulating interaction between the body and the air of the environment in three ways: through inhalation and exhalation; by opening and closing the pores of the skin; and by producing and maintaining the Defensive Qi. Because purified Qi of inhaled air is involved in the production of blood, the Lungs are involved in nutrition. Because inhalation sends water to the Kidneys, the Lung function also affects fluid balance in the body.

-Purifying inhaled air

The most important, and perhaps most apparent, function of the Lungs is to extract clean Qi from inhaled air. This purified essence of the air is combined with food essence from the Spleen, and sent it to the Heart where it becomes blood.

-Producing Defensive Qi

The Lungs produce the very important Wei Qi, or Defensive Qi, which is the body's first line of defense against pathogens from the environment. Wei Qi is closely related to the health of the skin and water metabolism (see below), particularly the opening and closing of the skin's pores. When Defensive Qi is weak, the body easily succumbs to attack from external pathogens, such as parasites and infectious pathogens.

- Activating the flow of Qi downward

Because the Lungs are the uppermost organs in the body, their Qi must descend. When it is not descending, such symptoms as coughing, asthmatic breathing, and stuffiness in the chest can occur. It can also cause shortness of breath, tiredness and drowsiness.

- Maintaining normal water metabolism

When the Lungs are functioning properly, inhalation will send water downward to the Kidney and Urinary Bladder. Failure of the water supply to these organs can result in dysuria (inability to urinate), edema (swelling), and/or phlegm-retention conditions.

The Lungs are also responsible for supplying the skin and hair with the body fluid they need to stay moist and bright. By spreading Qi between the muscles and the skin, the Lungs regulate the opening and closing of the skin's pores and keep the muscles warm. As part of the immune system, healthy skin defends the body from outside pathogenic factors. Unhealthy skin is associated with symptoms such as profuse sweating and vulnerability to the common cold.

METAL ELEMENT IMBALANCE

>>Physical signs:

- Shoulders rolled forward
- Phlegm
- Chronic coughing
- Dry skin (eczema)
- Stools dry and hard or loose
- Aversion to cold or heat
- Easily catches colds or flu

>>Emotional signs:

- Lack of willpower
- Disinclination to talk
- Lack of assertiveness
- Feelings of sadness, disappointment or despair
- Hypersensitivity
- Feeling exposed, vulnerable
- Unable to attain one's goals

PATH OF THE LUNG MERIDIAN

This meridian starts at the region of the stomach, moves down to connect with the large intestine, then rises back up through the diaphragm to the lungs. It continues up to the middle of each side of the collarbone, then out to each arm, passing in front of the bicep muscle, the center area of the elbow crease, the wrist, to the thumb pad. The meridian finishes at the outer side of base of the thumbnail.

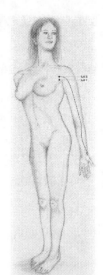

USEFUL ACUPOINTS ON THE LUNG MERIDIAN

LU1 & 2: These two points are very close to each other, at the tip of the crease when you bend your arm at the elbow. When you have phlegm, or a cough that produces phlegm, vigorously massage these points to warm them up.

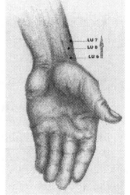

LU7, 8 & 9: These points are located at the wrist crease on the radial artery. Rubbing or massaging these points can help reduce a fever and/or subdue a cough, especially in children. For more thorough stimulation of the Lung meridian, starting at the wrist crease, vigorously rub the inside of the entire arm from wrist to elbow.

LUNG CLEANSING EXERCISE

This exercise particularly clears and harmonizes the energy of the Lung. It is useful for reducing any of the physical or emotional complaints listed above, or it may be used as a general health practice. It is particularly beneficial during the autumn to help strengthen the lungs. It can also help release excess sadness and sorrow.

THE MOVEMENT

1. Start with the Three Regulations: Steady breath, relaxed mind, Wu Ji posture (feet shoulder width, shoulders relaxed and broad, tailbone tucked, Crown Point rising). The tongue should be lightly touching the roof of the mouth behind the upper teeth.

2. Pull Down the Heavens three times.

3. With the eyes gazing forward, allow the arms to float up in front of the body to shoulder height, palms facing down.

4. While inhaling, spread the arms out to the side, palms down, as though opening curtains. This movement expands the chest.

5. Turn your palms up and, while exhaling, bring your arms back to the front, to the center of your body, closing your chest.

6. Repeat, with a continuous flowing motion.

7. End by Pulling Down the Heavens three times.

NOTES

1. It is recommended to do this 3-6 times for health maintenance; 9-36 times when addressing a particular problem.

2. You may enhance the efficacy of this exercise by saying the Lung sound "SSS" when exhaling.

CASE HISTORY

A two-year old baby had several seizures, which were terrifying for the parents. Their Western physician predicted that after a child has one seizure he is likely to have more by age 5 or 6, and he offered no preventative measures. The parents refused to accept this prediction, believing something could be done. They took the infant to an acupuncturist who prescribed an herbal formula to improve the baby's digestion. He also taught the parents to open the baby's arms in the Lung Movement and advised them to rub the baby's wrist and arm along the Lung Meridian. The parents reported that the baby never had another seizure.

Chapter 10: WATER ELEMENT

Yin Organ:	**Kidney**	**Hours: 5-7 pm**
Yang Organ:	**Urinary Bladder**	**Hours: 3-5 pm**

The Water Element relates to the Kidneys and the Urinary Bladder. It controls the skeletal system (bones), reproductive system including the testes and ovaries, and endocrine system including the adrenals, pancreas, hypothalamus, thyroid, pituitary gland, pineal gland, and thymus. Thus, the Kidneys rule overall constitution, health, and longevity. The health of the Kidneys is considered the foundation for the overall balance of all the other internal organs. The Yin aspect of the kidneys is storing the Essence of Life (Jing) and water; the Yang aspect is serving as the "life gate of fire", that is, as the motive force for transformation in the body. Because of these fundamental functions, the Kidneys are affected by any chronic disease.

The Kidneys rule the bones and produce bone marrow; the teeth are considered a surplus of the bones. The Kidneys open into the ears and the hair on the head. The ancient texts say that if the ears and Kidneys are harmonized, the ear can hear five tones. The moistness and vitality of the hair on the head are related to the Kidney essence. (The hair also depends on blood for nourishment which is why the hair on the head is also referred to as a surplus of blood.)

Kidney functions

The main functions of the Kidney are storing the Essence of Life, regulating water metabolism, and controlling and promoting inhalation.

- Storing the Essence of Life

There are two components of the Essence of Life. The first is known as the Prenatal Essence of Life, or Prenatal Qi. It is given at conception. It can be somewhat strengthened through food and nutrition, and is, or can be, transformed to the Qi of the Kidney. The Qi of the Kidney contributes to the growth, development, and replacement of the body, for example, the growth of teeth. The body grows as the Qi increases. When the body reaches puberty, the Qi of the Kidney is at its peak. It then initiates the production of sperm in boys and eggs and menstruation in girls. As the body ages, the Qi of the Kidney weakens, also diminishing reproductive capabilities.

The second component or type of Essence of Life is known as the acquired, or Postnatal, Qi. It is derived from food. The Spleen and the Stomach transform food into Postnatal Qi, which is then transported to the five viscera and six bowels. When there is not enough Postnatal Qi for body function, the Kidney will supply it from its reservoir; conversely, when there is surplus , the Kidney stores it. So, when any organ is not functioning correctly, the Kidney needs to be nourished because it will be relied upon to supply any deficiencies.

The Kidney's Essence of Life can aid in making bone marrow, which nourishes the bones. When the Kidney is functioning well, bones and teeth are strong. Conversely, when the Kidney is weak, both bones and teeth are weak also. The Essence of Life also turns into blood, which nourishes the hair. When the Kidney is functioning well, the hair is strong and shiny. Withered, balding, or gray hair can be a sign of a weak Kidney. Finally, the Kidneys also influence brain function; when Kidney Qi is strong, thinking and memory will also be strong and clear.

- Regulating water metabolism

The Kidney maintains balance of the fluid in the body. Fluid in the body is responsible for transporting nutrients to organs and tissues, and for carrying waste out of the tissues. The Kidney plays an important part in both functions. The Kidney either releases water or retains needed water. When the Kidney is functioning well, urination is normal. When it doesn't function well, the Kidney could release too much, causing diseases like polyuria (excess urination) and frequent urination. When the Kidney does not release enough, it can lead to oliguria (scant urination) and edema (swelling, excess water collecting in body tissues).

- Controlling and promoting respiration

According to Chinese medicine, the Kidney, along with the Lungs, aids in inhaling air. When the Kidney is not functioning well, exhaling will occur more than inhaling, which can result in dyspnea (difficult or labored breathing) and severe panting.

Kidney dysfunctions

In Chinese medical theory, Kidney Essence is like the battery power that runs your life. You can never have too much, but you can use it up. Thus, all Kidney disease patterns involve deficiency of some sort. Sources of potential deficiencies—that is, ways your Kidney Essence can become exhausted-- fall into six categories: Hereditary, emotional, sexual, chronic illness, aging, and overwork.

- Hereditary weakness

Prenatal Qi or Life Essence is formed at conception; its quality is determined by the quality of the parents' Essences, Heavenly Qi, and the environment. If the parents' Essences are weak, which means they had weak constitutions, then the child will also be weak and may have such symptoms as poor bone development, poor teeth, enuresis (inability to hold urine), thin or weak hair, and in extreme cases some mental retardation. Since a person's vital energy naturally declines with age, conceiving late in life can weaken the constitution of the child. When Prenatal Qi is weak, the person must pay particular attention to the other factors in order not to put a stress, or drain, on this irreplaceable vital force.

- Emotions

Fear, fright, shock, and anxiety makes the Qi descend, especially in children. It can happen to anybody; something that happens to you or something that you witness can cause shock, and deplete your Kidney Qi. In adults such depletion may be the root cause for insomnia and mental restlessness.

- Sexual activity

Excess of sexual orgasms weakens the Kidneys because orgasms are directly related to the Kidney Essence. This also includes masturbation. Since the Heart and Kidneys are closely related, during an orgasm one can often experience palpitations. Conversely, Heart deficiency caused by sadness and anxiety can weaken the Kidneys and cause impotence or lack of sex drive, as well as coldness in the limbs and enuresis (involuntary urination).

- Chronic illness

Any long-lasting, chronic condition will create a deficiency of Kidney Yang and/or Kidney Yin.

- Aging

Kidney Essence naturally declines with age. In fact, in Chinese medicine the process of aging is defined as the manifestation of a decrease of the Kidney Essence. Hence, as a person ages, they experience decline in all the functions controlled by Kidney Essence, namely, decreases in hearing, bone density, sexual function, memory, and hair.

- Overwork

This means mental and physical work for long periods of time or burning the candles at both ends. In modern society, this is the most common cause of depleted Kidney Yin. Long work hours, particularly mental work, in poor environments, emotional stress, lack of relaxation, lack of exercise, improper and irregular meals, poor sleep, lack of exercise, etc. draws directly on Yang energy. When Yang energy normally used for these functions is exhausted, the body starts using the Yin Essence. Yin Essence is generally harder to restore, and its depletion leads to problems that are more difficult to treat. In all of these cases, eliminating the drain on Yang Essence is the first step to recovery.

WATER ELEMENT IMBALANCE

>>Physical signs:

- Arthritis
- Poor memory
- Ringing of the ears
- Bone degeneration
- Premature hair loss and or graying
- Involuntary loss of semen
- Lack of sex drive
- Infertility
- Shortness of breath
- Hearing loss
- Too little or too much urination

>>Emotional signs:

- ☯ Lack of motivation and drive; apathy
- ☯ Being fearful or apprehensive
- ☯ Inability to confront issues
- ☯ Inertia

PATH OF THE KIDNEY MERIDIAN

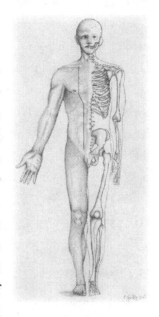

The Kidney Meridian starts underneath the base of the small toe, moves over to the center of the foot at the base of the ball of the foot, then runs across the sole, emerging along the arch. It circles the inner ankle, then ascends along the inside of the lower leg, behind both the Liver and Spleen meridians, to the inner knee crease. It continues on the inside of the thigh, and then enters the torso near the base of the spine. One branch connects internally with the Kidneys and Bladder. From there it emerges to the surface of the abdomen above the pubic bone, runs upward over the abdomen and chest, and ends at the collar bone . Another internal branch ascends to connect with the Liver, Lung, Heart, and ends at the base of the tongue.

USEFUL ACUPOINTS

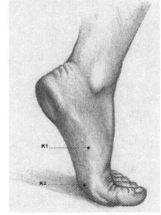

K1: This point is known as the Bubbling Spring point. It is located in the center of the ball of the foot. Pat it with a cupped hand for insomnia due to an overactive mind. It is also good to rub to relieve shock, as of an accident. Or, to relieve a cold, rub liniment oil into the point and then go to bed.

K2: This point is located on the inner side, or instep, of the foot, where the bulge of the big toe starts. Massage this point to tonify the body or to relieve aching feet. It may also be used for problems of the reproductive system, such as infertility or nocturnal emissions.

KIDNEY CLEANSING EXERCISE

This exercise particularly clears and harmonizes the energy of the Kidney. Use it to relieve any of the physical or emotional symptoms listed above. Or use it as part of a general health routine.

THE MOVEMENT

1. Start with the Three Regulations: Steady breath, relaxed mind, Wu Ji posture (feet shoulders' width, shoulders relaxed and broad, tailbone tucked, Crown Point rising).

2. Pull Down the Heavens three times.

3. Roll the tip of the tongue back to the soft palate on the roof of the mouth.

4. Place the back of the left hand on the lower back, in the region of the right kidney.

5. Bring the right arm up to the left side of the body, about eye level, palm outward.

6. Inhale as you sweep your arm to the right, gazing at the back of the right arm..

7. Then exhale as you bend forward at the waist, and scooping with your right arm in front of your body from right to left.

8. Continuing this as a circular motion. That is, inhale as you sweep your arm, at eye level, to the right, then exhale as you scoop/sweep your arm to the left at knee level.

9. Repeat several times, then switch and do the same exercise on the left side.

10. Finish by Pulling Down the Heavens three times.

NOTES

1. As part of a daily health routine, repeat 3x on each side. When targeting a specific problem, repeat it 9-36 x on each side.

2. To increase the efficacy of the exercise, you may say the Kidney sound, "FUUU", when exhaling. The "U" is pronounced as "oo"

3. The left Kidney represents Kidney Yin while the right represents Kidney Yang, which is the motive force for heat and transformation in the body. Thus, it is important to do both sides equally.

CASE HISTORY

A client had a flu bug that had lasted for eight months; we call this a "febrile disease" as it involved a low-grade fever in the body. Her Western physician had not been able to help her recover. She saw a Chinese doctor who prescribed herbs and gave her acupressure. This cured the flu, but she then developed a chronic case of vertigo (Meniere's Disease). Again, the Western physician couldn't help. When she came to me, I assessed the problem as a depletion of Kidney Essence. I gave her moxa (a warming treatment) and acupuncture on specific Kidney points. Her homework was to do the Kidney Movement daily, and particularly whenever she had an incidence of vertigo. Within a week she saw improvement; within 4-6 weeks all her symptoms were gone.

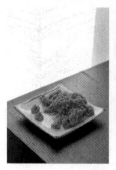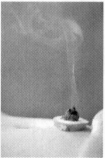

Chapter 11: WOOD ELEMENT

Yin Organ:	**Liver**	**Hours: 1-3 am**	
Yang Organ:	**Gall Bladder**	**Hours: 11 pm-1 am**	

In the Chinese system, the Wood Element corresponds to the Liver and Gall Bladder energies in the human body. Anatomically, the liver organ is located in the upper right part of the abdomen, behind the lower part of the rib cage. In Chinese medicine, the main functions of the Liver concern filtering, storing and regulating blood and regulating Qi. The quality of Liver energy is specifically reflected in the quality of the tendons, ligaments, sinews, nails and eyes.

In Chinese medicine, the Liver is often compared to trees, as both tend to "spread out freely". The Liver's function is to spread Qi throughout the body. It accomplishes this in three ways: regulating mind and mood, promoting digestion and absorption, and keeping Qi and blood moving normally. In Chinese medicine, the Heart and Liver regulate the flow of vital energy and blood, which results in an even temper, feelings of happiness, and relaxation. But when the Liver does not function well, it results in anxiety, irritability, anger and resentment. Modern society places particular stress on the Liver, both in the type of food we eat and the stresses inherent in daily life. Road rage is a typical example of Liver Qi imbalance, in a Chinese doctor's terms.

The Liver's function of regulating the flow of energy in the body also specifically aids the Spleen in distributing nutrients and water in the body, and therefore, contributes to good digestion. An unhealthy Liver can affect the Spleen negatively, resulting in poor appetite, belching, vomiting, and diarrhea.

The Liver's function of regulating the flow of energy directly affects the flow of blood. Erratic blood flow can result in symptoms throughout the lower abdomen, in particular for women, affecting the menstrual blood.

WOOD ELEMENT IMBALANCE

>>Physical signs:

- ☯ Floaters or blurred vision
- ☯ Eye or facial tremors
- ☯ Unsettled sleep, especially waking between 1-3 am
- ☯ Menstrual irregularities, especially blocked or reduced flow
- ☯ Hypochondria pain (i.e., pain just below the ribs)
- ☯ Chemical sensitivities
- ☯ Uneven energy throughout the day
- ☯ Migraine headaches
- ☯ Constipation
- ☯ Nausea

>>Emotional signs:

- ☯ Depression
- ☯ Sudden outbursts or feelings of overwhelming rage and anger
- ☯ Inability to handle stressful situations

PATH OF THE LIVER MERIDIAN

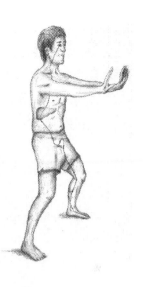

The Liver Meridian begins at the pinky side of the big toenail. It then goes over the top of the foot, in front of the inner ankle, along the inner side of the shin bone, and up past the knee. It continues up the inner side of the thigh to the pubic region where it encircles the genitalia before entering the lower abdomen and ascending to the liver and gall bladder. It then spreads across the diaphragm and ribs, ascends to the neck, throat, and eye system, and ends at the top of the head.

USEFUL ACUPOINTS ON THE LIVER MERIDIAN

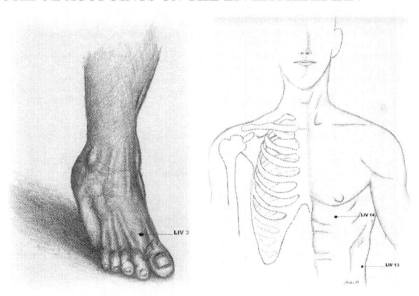

LIV3: This point is located on the top of the foot, between the tendons leading to the big toe and the next toe. It can be used to drain excess energy from the Liver Channel; if it is painful when touched, then massage will help any symptom resulting from excess Liver energy. Use this for

acute attacks of anger, or massage regularly for harmonizing menstrual irregularities, disturbed sleep, eye problems, etc.

LIV13: This point is located on the top of the floating ribs, on both sides of the body, below the armpit. Massage this point when you have a 'stitch' in your side, for depression, or to help control function of the gall bladder and spleen.

LIV14: This point is located below each nipple in the spaces between the ribs. It connects directly with the liver, and massaging it can help reduce intense feelings of anger or resentment. (This is a point that is tender to the touch for most people.)

LIVER CLEANSING EXERCISE

This exercise particularly clears and harmonizes the energy of the liver. It is useful for reducing any of the physical or emotional complaints listed above. On the emotional level, it targets and reduces the negative emotions of anger and frustration, while encouraging kindness and compassion.

THE MOVEMENT

1. Start with the Three Regulations: Steady breath, relaxed mind, Wu Ji posture (feet shoulder width apart, shoulders relaxed and broad, tailbone tucked, Crown Point rising). The tongue should be pointing straight up, touching the roof of the mouth.

2. Pull Down the Heavens three times.

3. Bring the right hand, palm up, to the right side of the body. Position it at the ribs.

4. Stretch the left hand forward, wrist cocked so the palm faces out, as if you were trying to push something away from the body.

5. Pull the left arm / palm back, as you push the right arm/palm out. The left palm pulls in to the left side of the ribs, facing up while the right arm extends forward, palm vertical, facing away from

you. In other words, the left hand goes back to where the right hand started and the right hand pushes out as the left hand initially did. Widen the eyes and stretch the tendons of the fingers of your outstretched hand.

6. Repeat this exchange. There should be a rolling effect of the palms as they pass one another midway through the movement.

7. Finish by Pulling Down the Heavens three times.

NOTES

1. Do this daily, to keep your Liver energy flowing smoothly, but particularly if you have issues to do with anger, resentment or frustration.

2. Keep your shoulders relaxed.

3. To increase the effect of the exercise, you may say the sound for the Liver, which is "SHUUU".

CASE HISTORY

A woman, who appeared to be very fit and who was a fitness trainer herself, came in with back problems. Reading her face, I saw signs of unresolved anger, which I suspected had created deep-seated regrets. She denied this, saying she had dealt with those issues; she believed that good diet and exercise were enough to maintain her health. Even so I suggested she should have a cardiovascular checkup. Reports showed that both carotid arteries were 76% blocked. She's now doing all the Yin organ exercises and sounds, with particular emphasis on those for the Liver and Heart. At the same time, she is working on her emotional health, spending time to become aware of and resolve issues. She says she realizes that emotions, as well as diet and exercise, are a critical component of overall health.

Chapter 12: STAYING PRESENT

You have now taken the first steps in establishing your Qigong practice. You have learned the White Pearl Meditation, which is particularly good for replenishing your life batteries, the Kidneys. You have learned the Center and Balance Meditation, a good technique for keeping yourself centered and grounded. You have learned to "Brush the Meridians", to keep energy flowing. You have some experience with the Micro-Cosmic Orbit, which will lead you deeper and deeper into awareness of the ebb and flow of Qi in your body. In addition you have learned five exercises to harmonize the key Yin organs, one for each of the Five Elements. Most important of all, I hope you have learned to be present with your body. The mental world constantly lures us, with hopes, fear, regrets, thoughts of past and future, but our life is here, now. Your body, your very own Qi, can be one of the most exciting parts of your universe.

I hope, too, that in doing these exercises you have experienced some benefit. Maybe not much, and maybe not every time, but enough to show you the value of them, and enough to make you want to continue. As with any other human activity, getting benefit demands that you DO IT. Ideally, regularly. In the next section I will describe three different daily routines—the full routine for those with time and dedication (1- 2 hours); the 20-minute routine; and the 1-minute routine. For everyone, I recommend doing the Renewal of Spirit Meditation (described later, here) every week on Sunday. As with every other part of the cosmos, our energies function rhythmically, cyclically. Yang energy begins to build from Sunday, peaking on Wednesday, then declining as Yin energy builds. Thus Sunday is that still point when we can pause, re-establish our center, and express our intention for the week. (It could also be a good day for working people to do the full routine that they can't manage on a weekday.) Create a routine that you can realistically manage, persevere with patience, and be confident that results are coming.

SUGGESTED DAILY ROUTINES

The Full Routine (1-2 hours)

1. Remembering the Three Regulations, assume the Wu Ji posture.

2. Pull Down the Heavens three times.

3. Do the three Body Awakening Exercises; finish by Pulling Down the Heavens.

4. Do the Center and Balance Meditation. (Do this until you can feel your whole body simultaneously. In the beginning this may take 10-14 minutes; later you will achieve the sensation in 1-2 minutes.) Pull Down the Heavens three times.

5. Do the Micro-Cosmic Orbit, 5-10 minutes. Pull Down the Heavens three times.

6. Brush the Meridians, three times; Pull Down the Heavens three times.

7. Massage the Yang Organs; Pull Down the Heavens three times.

8. Do the preparation move for the Five Yin Organ Exercises; then do each of the Yin Organ exercises, beginning with the Heart, the Emperor of the body. Do each one at least three times; you may do more for any Organ that you want to target. Pull Down the Heavens three times.

9. Finish with the White Pearl Meditation, storing all the Essence you have gathered in your battery pack, the Kidneys.

20-Minute Routine

1. Remembering the Three Regulations, assume the Wu Ji posture.

2. Pull Down the Heavens three times.

3. Do the three Body Awakening Exercises; finish by Pulling Down the Heavens.

4. Do the Micro-Cosmic Orbit, 5-10 minutes. Pull Down the Heavens three times.

5. Do the preparation move for the Five Yin Organ Exercises; then do each of the Yin Organ exercises, beginning with the Heart, the Emperor of the body. Do each one at least three times; you may do more for any Organ that you want to target. Pull Down the Heavens three times.

6. Finish with the White Pearl Meditation, storing all the Essence you have gathered in your battery pack, the Kidneys.

One-Minute Routine

1. Remembering the Three Regulations, assume the Wu Ji posture.

2. Pull Down the Heavens three times.

3. Do the White Pearl Meditation.

4. Pull Down the Heavens three times.

RENEWAL OF SPIRIT MEDITATION

This meditation can be done daily or once a week, ideally on Sundays, to renew your Qi for the week. It is also ideal to do during any seasonal change such as the spring or vernal equinox. You can start with invocations, prayer and/or an energy cultivation practice, or simply begin.

1. As usual, start with the Three Regulations: Steady breath, relaxed mind, Wu Ji posture (feet shoulder width, shoulders relaxed and broad, tailbone tucked, Crown Point rising).

2. Pull Down the Heavens three times.

3. Allow heavenly energy to descend. As this divine Qi descends, imagine that any and all dark turbid Qi from the body is pushed out through the feet, deep into the earth.

4. Start doing the Mystical Pearl Meditation: Focusing on your breathing, breathe deeply into the lower Dan Tian for five minutes. Imagine the Dan Tian filling with golden mystical light from the Earth.

5. Now bring your awareness to the Third Eye, the center of the forehead, the Upper Dan Tian, and imagine a brown pearl turning there. Feel this brown pearl pulsating, rotating, vibrating.

6. Next imagine peeling away the brown skin of this pearl, then polishing it until it is brilliant white, shining and filling the entire Upper Dan Tian with pure radiance, illuminating all your senses.

7. Next imagine that the white light descends through your body, cleansing everything in its path.

8. Now focus on the golden light of the Lower Dan Tian and allow the golden and white lights to mix. Feel the mixed energy cleansing every part of your body, both physical and emotional.

9. Imagine the cleansing energy moving down. Focus on the bottoms of the feet and imagine turbid energy leaving through the base of the balls of the feet, replaced by pure energy.

10. As you feel your body becoming purified, cleansed, and rejuvenated, start to bring your awareness back to the present.

11. Slowly awaken all your sensory organs one at a time. Start with your ears, allowing for a complete opening of the ears. Next, stimulate your saliva and the mouth, allowing for the mouth to fully awaken. Then awaken the nose, allowing for the senses of your nose to bring in positive life force energy.

12. Finally the pores of the skin: Allow the pores to open, bringing you heightened awareness of everything around you. Feel your environment and your connectedness to everything.

13. Now, simply, relax. You are ready to start your day (week) with increased awareness, alertness, and profound tranquility, grounded and centered in your true nature.

14. Pull Down the Heavens three times, just for good measure.

Chapter 13: THE FIVE ELEMENT QUESTIONNAIRE

Like other aspects of the world, our own personalities can be understood in terms of the Five Elements. The Elements are expressed in what we look like, how we act, how we feel—and they can be used to predict what diseases we are likely to suffer from. Knowing the strengths and weaknesses of the Elements in your nature can help you understand yourself better and help you make life-affirming choices in every sphere of life from diet to home décor. More broadly, recognizing Element archetypes in others can help you understand the people you meet on a deeper, more compassionate level.

In the Appendix you will find a Five Element Questionnaire. Take this Questionnaire now to assess your personality in terms of the Five Elements. Are you a Wood Type? Fire Type? Or a mixture of two? Are you a Fire Type with Metal issues? In future lessons we will discuss each of the five archetypes in depth. First, simply take the Questionnaire.

Instructions for taking the Questionnaire: The questions are grouped in five sections, or "phases". Answer according to how you are now—not how you want to be, or how you used to be. If the condition in the question sounds a lot like you, put a +2. If the condition (or attitude) sounds somewhat like you, put a +1. Conversely, if the question doesn't describe you at all, put -2, or, if somewhat, then -1. Put a 0 for neutral. Do not get caught up in the details, especially whether it's -1 or -2. Later, in evaluating your scores, you will be interested in their spread—that is, what are the highest and lowest scores-- not in what is in between.

When you have answered all the questions, add up the count for each phase. Arrange the phases in order from highest score to lowest score. Turn to the Five Element Questionnaire Answers in the Appendix to learn which phase corresponds to which Element.

Advice for interpreting your results: This questionnaire will reveal the predominant (highest score) and weakest (lowest score) archetypes, or Elements, in your personality. At the beginning, for the sake of keeping things simple, concern yourself only with your predominant and weakest Elements. It is possible that your predominant type is a combination--a Metal/Earth type for example—but don't consider that possibility at first.

Your highest score/strongest archetype describes the fundamental way you approach the world. Deviations from your predominant archetype may explain why certain personality traits, habits, and/or health issues bother you. Your lowest score suggests areas of weakness where you might want to focus energy to achieve more balance and harmony. The descriptions of the individual archetypes in later chapters will guide you in understanding how to do this.

Many factors--including diet, where you live, the way that you live your life, the type of friends you choose, etc.--can create variations to these archetypes. These factors can also influence whether the archetype is expressed in a positive or negative way. Remember, too, that your fundamental archetype may change with different stages in your life.

Chapter 14: FIRE ARCHETYPE

Compass direction: South

Season: Summer

Color: Red

Taste: Bitter

Internal organs: Heart, Small Intestine; Pericardium; Triple Warmer

Expressed in: Eyes

Positive expressions: Joy, clarity, love

Negative emotions: Sadness, confusion, over-excitation, manic behavior

Underlying principle

The Fire Element, most active in the summer, represents exuberant activity, warmth, and clarity.

Physical attributes

Fire people tend to be small in stature with slim hips and shoulders, mobile hands, sparkling eyes and redness in the throat and neck areas. Lively, cute, and charming, their main goal in life is to play. They love new experiences and excitement; they can become thrill seekers. They bask in the limelight, and are generally charismatic, charming, and adept at communication. They are full of ideas but prefer starting to finishing. To a more sedate personality, the Fire person can appear impulsive, changeable and scattered. The Fire type is normally unconcerned with wealth, yet fond of beauty. They are naturally attuned to rhythm and love to dance to a strong beat. Fire minds can be so active that they never shut down, and this can lead to elaborate and active dreams. A Fire type can illuminate and give comfort in any situation. This archetype tends to walk fast, be very creative, and willingly take on many challenges. They tend to flourish in warmer climates as they dislike wearing much clothing and have a naturally high body temperature.

The Fire Element rules the Heart, which in turn is considered to rule the expression of all emotions. Even though every organ has its own emotions, the Heart decides whether the emotion is to be expressed and to what extent. The Fire Element governs communications of all kinds, especially the use of words spoken verbally or in sign language with the hands. Because the Heart controls expression, the wrinkles on the face show how much expression has been used over time. The ancient Chinese feared Fire because, in excess, it dries up the all-important Yin essence and wears out the body. However, Fire is also so necessary to the enjoyment of life that containing it too much may be even more harmful. There is a primal human need for expression and enjoyment.

The strength of Fire is shown—is said to "burn"-- in the tips and the corners of all the facial features. Sharp tips of the eyebrows, ears, nose, lips, and a pointed chin are all Fire traits. Fire also "burns" particularly in the eyes. The eyes are the facial feature most closely associated with this Element. Their brightness and quality reflect the quality of inner spirit, or *shen*. From the *shen*, you can determine how quick someone's mind is. Babies with bright eyes are recognized as very intelligent. The *shen* also shows the changes in emotion from moment to moment, and reflects how well the nervous system is functioning. Because of the complex network of muscles that surround the eyes, they are the most expressive feature on the face and the most easily marked. We learn very early in life how to communicate with our eyes, and they reveal our inner truths.

Emotional attributes

The emotions that are particularly associated with the heart are joy and sadness. Practitioners of Chinese medicine today often talk of "excess joy" being dangerous. I believe that this is a mistranslation. What the ancients really meant was that excess excitement or mania, not joy, was considered harmful to the health. Also, somewhat in contradiction to typical interpretations, I consider sadness an emotion of the Heart, not of the Lungs. Sadness is just the letdown from the high that Fire lives on. It is the period between the time when the candle flame blows out and when it is relit. Because the Heart and Lungs are closely connected, sadness can turn into sorrow, which is definitely a Lung emotion. In time, unless resolved, the sorrow becomes grief, the primary Lung emotion.

Recognizing disharmonies in the Fire Element

>Strong Fire

If your score shows that you are primarily a Fire type then look to the blood and blood vessels, and to the nervous system, for keys to your physical health. A Fire type's most serious health problems are likely to come from inflammation, which is caused by unrestrained Fire and an overactive nervous system. This includes lupus and rheumatoid arthritis. Fire people are also prone to disturbances in speaking and thinking that are caused by misfiring of the brain and overactive imaginations. These include stuttering, phobias, and mental illnesses. The Fire Element's primary organ is the Heart, which controls and regulates the expression of all emotions. Suppression of emotions can therefore cause problems with the heart including arrhythmia, tachycardia and heart disease. Fire people maintain a youthful persona and try to continue living an erratic life that ultimately leads to burnout and sadness.

>Deficient Fire

People who are deficient in the Fire Element may be prone to heart-related problems, and/or problems with their veins, arteries, and/or blood.

Achieving harmony in the Fire Element

To increase the power of the Fire Element in your life, use the color red, angular objects, and anything bright and shining in decorating your living space. For example, you may want to wear more red in your clothes or add candles, pictures containing fire or pictures of buildings with steep roofs, like churches steeples to your environment. Pyramid shapes and mountain ranges with steep peaks also support the Fire aspect. Sleeping with your head in the south will also increase the influence of Fire.

Conversely, to calm overactive Fire reduce all these influences. Also, consider adding calming practices such as yoga and meditation and limiting your social life to give your internal batteries a chance to recharge.

In terms of diet, the Fire person should avoid alcoholic beverages and caffeine, both of which would exacerbate the active principle. Adding bitter foods, particularly those that grow quickly such as kale, dandelion greens, bitter lettuces such as escarole, as well as other bitter foods, such as bitter melon, would be very beneficial as the bitter flavor stimulates flow of energy in the Heart meridian.

CASE HISTORY

At a certain point in my life, I knew my Fire Element was deficient in Qi. Several relationships had ended badly; I felt discouraged and frustrated. My heart center was unwilling to invest in another relationship, yet I craved companionship. To restore my heart Fire, I changed my living environment. I shifted my bed so that, when sleeping, my head would be in the South. I bought two red pyramids (a shape that represents Fire) and placed them on the windowsill above the bed. I also added red items to the room's décor, for example, red candles. The effects were not instant, but over a 1-2 month period I noticed changes. I met more Fire people, and felt more optimistic. Ultimately it was at this time I met my current partner, who is a Fire type.

Chapter 15: EARTH ARCHETYPE

Compass direction: Central

Season: Late summer/Early autumn

Color: Yellow

Taste: Sweet

Internal organs: Spleen, Stomach

Expressed in: Muscles, mouth (lips)

Positive expressions: Serenity, centeredness, affection

Negative emotions: Worry, anxiety

Underlying principle

The Earth Element, most active in the late summer/early autumn, represents stability, serenity, and warm affection.

Physical attributes

The major physical signs of Earth are plumpness in the abdominal area, lower cheeks of the face, upper arms and calves. The Earth archetype may have a darkish complexion, strong thighs, and wide jaws. In particular, Earth types should have strong muscles. The Earth person has to watch out for gaining weight, because a large belly and somewhat fat body are attributes of the Earth type.

The facial feature most strongly related to the Earth Element is the mouth, particularly the lips. The mouth is the place to take in nourishment and is also the most sensual part of the face. The size of the mouth shows the appetite, not only for food but also for affection, information, things, etc. The bigger the mouth, the more a person wants. The mouth is a feature that expresses emotions easily, with a smile or a kiss. It is the second most changeable feature on the face, after the eyes. Most major expressions require movement of the mouth. The mobility of the muscles around the mouth allows people to change its shape in an extraordinary range.

A large mouth shows generosity and the ability to give. Larger mouths belong to people who have lots of Earth energy. Mouth size is measured in relation to the nose. Imagine a triangle starting at the center point in the bridge of the nose and follow the sides of the nose down to the mouth area. The average mouth is the same length as the width at the base of this imaginary triangle. Any mouth that goes beyond this measurement is considered wide. Any mouth smaller than this measurement can be considered small.

To the ancient Chinese, a large mouth was considered a fortunate feature. Men with large mouths are supposedly more capable of getting a good wife. People with large mouths are typically generous, for example, buying many gifts for people they love as well as for business associates. They can be known to spontaneously give things even to strangers or new acquaintances. People with average-sized mouths still have generosity but are more particular about to whom and how much they give. People with small mouths find it difficult to give unless there is a good reason. They are more conditional about their giving. They give because someone deserves it or because they are supposed to give something; they give based on practicality more than emotion.

The size of the lips is also a factor. Fullness of the lips is evaluated based on the fleshiness of the rest of the face. Someone whose face is earthier, with plump cheeks and a puffy nose will have bigger lips. Someone whose skin is taut with aquiline features will have thinner lips. Exceptions to this are magnified traits. In general, fuller lips belong to people who are more expressive emotionally. They are romantic and sensual. These lips indicate a desire for pleasure. People with thinner lips are more reserved emotionally, especially if they hold them compressed.

Vertical wrinkles on the philtrum above the upper lip can indicate Earth deficiency, or conditions where the person typically gives more than he/she receives, or has somehow not been nurtured fully through their lives. It also can reflect a deficiency in physical nutrition.

Emotional attributes

Earth people tend to be sedentary; they enjoy sitting. They value comfort, consistency and pleasure. They thoroughly enjoy food and companionship. They are the collectors of the world and love to accumulate possessions and people. They become very attached to their things and loved ones. They are generally considered warm and affectionate.

Although not ambitious, Earth types are calm and centered. Earth represents stability, and the Element harmonizes all other Elements. Being fair is a predominant quality of Earth types. As they can be trusted, they make great managers and organizers. At the same time, their focus can be weak, making handling multiple tasks very difficult, and they tend to worry. They respond to change well as long as it is gradual.

Recognizing disharmonies in the Earth Element

>Strong Earth

When the Earth Element is in excess, there is a strong tendency to overeat and gain weight to the point of obesity. Earth people tend to worry and feel excess sympathy for those they care about. This can lead them to become overly involved in the lives of others. As Earth people move slowly, they can get stuck in habits, creating cycles and patterns that are hard to shift.

>Stagnant Earth

Earth stagnation is shown in the tendency for the circulation of the lymph fluid and blood to pool or coagulate causing such problems as varicose veins, blood clots and hemorrhoids.

>Deficient Earth

When the Earth Element is deficient, there are problems with the stomach and the ingestion and digestion of food—as well as ideas. Related conditions include anorexia, bulimia, diabetes, and flatulence. Earth deficiency is common when too much nurturing is given to others at the expense of the self. This is thought to be an underlying causative emotional factor in cancer. Movement and change is to be encouraged for a more balanced Earth Element.

Achieving harmony in the Earth Element

The colors yellow, orange, and earth tones support the Earth Element. To benefit this Element hang pictures of flat lands or plains. The Earth Element is represented by architecture that is both flat and square. Having your surroundings made of earth-derived building materials, which include brick, adobe, or even concrete, is positive for supporting earth.

While Earth types may be attracted to sugars and sweets, they should avoid excessive amounts of simple carbohydrates. Foods that may help uplift fatigue caused by weakness are yams, corn, and certain types of rice. People that need to balance their Earth Element will greatly benefit from Qigong practices that help root the Qi, and practices that help harmonize the Stomach and Spleen. They will also benefit from hobbies that help them regain their sense of being grounded, such as working with clay, gardening, or simply spending time outdoors in nature.

As the sweet flavor is associated with Earth, those deficient in Earth could add more sweet, yellow or orange foods to their diet, and should eat more bland foods like oatmeal or rice porridge. Conversely, those seeking to harmonize excess Earth should avoid these foods.

Chapter 16: METAL ARCHETYPE

Compass direction: West

Season: Autumn

Color: White

Taste: Pungent

Internal organs: Lungs, Large Intestine

Expressed in: Hair, skin

Positive expressions: Courage, righteousness, justice, truth

Negative emotions: Grief, sorrow, sadness, disappointment

Underlying principle

The Metal Element, most active in the autumn, represents the principles of independence, correctness, and sensitivity on all levels.

Physical attributes

The major signs of Metal are small bones, very fair skin and aquiline features. While perhaps appearing delicate, they typically have strong bodies with broad, square shoulders. They may walk slowly, pushing their chest out with their shoulders back.

Metal people have very strong immune systems; they can get sick frequently, but recover quickly. People who are Metal types typically develop skin and respiratory system allergies early in life including hives, eczema and asthma. Metal types get sunburned easily, and prefer staying indoors. They are more easily bitten by mosquitoes because of their ability to release a large quantity of carbon dioxide with their out-breath as they detoxify their lungs. They prefer to cocoon in what they consider safe environments with a minimum of dust or clutter and a maximum of beauty and stylish design.

In addition to the fine-boned structure and white undertone to the complexion, the facial feature that most strongly expresses the Metal Element is the nose.

Emotional attributes

Metal types are typically more mental than physical. They require refinement, cleanliness, tranquility and space to thrive. Metaphorically, the Element encompasses both people who are like raw ore, out of the earth--practical, independent, strong-willed--and people who are like fine, honed steel—elegant, sensitive, idealistic. Hence, Metal types can love both simplicity and luxury. They are particular, detail-oriented and perfectionist. Metal people normally have strong voices, their lungs being their strongest attribute. They also express strong voice in being aggressive in pursuing their goals, confident, and intuitive. They are as sensitive to dust and clutter as they are to injustice and dishonesty; they demand respect.

In their negative aspect, Metal types are often seen as aloof and distant, and, indeed, they may isolate themselves, withdrawing from activities and society in general, but this could express their need to maintain their boundaries as they easily get overwhelmed. Metal types are prone to health problems involving violation of their boundaries and/or failure to express their inner feelings. In Chinese Medicine, the emotion of sorrow is typically associated with the Lungs and Metal Element. This could arrive from the fact that the deepest sorrow derives from separation from those you love, either by death or by behavior. The correlations presented here suggest that breathing deeply may be one of the best self-help methods for restoring a balanced view and acceptance of circumstances causing sorrow.

Recognizing disharmonies in the Metal Element

> Strong Metal

When Metal is too strong, a person becomes rigid and inflexible, with emotional as well as physical repercussions. Phobias may develop.

> Stagnant Metal

Conditions of stagnation include illnesses that occur because of overcrowding and unclean environments including tuberculosis and leprosy. Excessive accumulation of phlegm that causes chronic coughing and shortness of breath are also associated with Metal stagnation.

> Deficient Metal

When people develop allergies later in life, they usually have become Metal deficient. This also applies to those who never got respiratory ailments as children but do suffer from them frequently as adults. Other signs of Metal deficiency include the slow healing of skin and chronic respiratory and skin conditions including recurring bronchitis, emphysema, psoriasis and weakening of the immune system. A tendency to catch colds or flus easily could be a sign of a weak Metal element.

Achieving harmony in the Metal Element

To support the Metal Element include metal items and furnishings in your life and house. Use the colors white or silver. Decorate your house with arched, curved, or semi-circular, furnishings to gather more Metal energy. In architecture, domed metal roofs or primarily metal structures attract Metal energy.

In terms of diet, to increase Metal Element, take pungent foods that expel pathogens from the body. Examples include garlic, ginger, and mint. All members of the cabbage family, including horseradish, can supply pungent flavor and support the immune system.

Chapter 17: WATER ARCHETYPE

Compass direction: North

Season: Winter

Color: Black or deep blue

Taste: Salty

Internal organs: Kidney, Urinary Bladder

Expressed in: Bones, ears, hair, brain, uterus/testicles

Positive expressions: Wisdom, insight

Negative emotions: Fear

Underlying principle

The Kidneys store the willpower. The Yang aspect of this will is the power to take responsibility for one's life, making decisive efforts and fundamental commitments. The Yin aspect is the recognition that the deepest force requires no work. The Yin will influences the direction in which we move; it can only be seen or noticed when we look back and realize how much we have developed over time. Through the interplay of these two, without fear, we develop wisdom.

Physical attributes

The major physical signs of Water are big bones or wide hips; Water people carry weight in their hips and thighs. They often look multiethnic which gives them an exotic, mysterious or secretive persona. They are prone to shadows around the eyes.

The facial features most strongly related to the Water Element are the ears, forehead, philtrum, chin, and under the eyes. The shape, size and quality of the tissue of your ears are indicative of the quality and strength of your Qi. A broad prominent forehead suggests creativity.

Emotional attributes

Water people are quiet and observant. They are good listeners and give good advice because they have innate wisdom. They appear to be easygoing, but when working, they are very persistent. They require a lot of sleep, rest, meditation or time to just "be". They are strong people both physically and emotionally. They handle catastrophes and emergencies calmly. They need to watch being too willful or stubborn. Their main health problems come from the frozen state of Water, which encourages growth of tumors or high blood pressure from the lack of flow of the emotions.

Recognizing disharmonies in the Water Element

>Strong Water

Strong Water energy usually leads to longevity when life is lived wisely and energy is conserved rather than spent. In Western terms this is often attributed to good genetic stock, which is indeed an important factor. Problems arising with the Water Element are typically diagnosed as either stagnant or deficient, never excess.

>Stagnant Water

When the Water energy stagnates, it is not accessible or usable, which affects the thinking and is implicated in mental illness and depression.

>Deficient Water

Deficient Water occurs when the lifestyle is too active and Qi is not replenished. This causes aging and degeneration of the body as well as problems with infertility and impotence. Water deficiency can be seen in the following conditions: loss of bone density, losing teeth, deafness, thinning hair, osteoarthritis and bladder weakness. Genetic defects are also considered a primary form of Water deficiency.

Achieving harmony in the Water Element

To enhance the Water Element, use dark blue or black colors and/or round bowl-shaped objects in your décor, fluid shapes and pictures of water—ideally active water, such as waterfalls rather than placid lakes, which can promote stagnation. Also the addition of a fountain or playing an audio track of flowing water will promote Water energy.

In terms of diet, adding dark colored and/or salty foods such as seaweeds, black beans, kidney beans, etc. can be very beneficial as the flavor stimulates flow of energy in the Kidney and Urinary Bladder meridians.

Chapter 18: WOOD ARCHETYPE

Compass direction: East

Season: Spring

Color: Green

Taste: Sour

Internal organs: Liver, Gall Bladder

Expressed in: Tendons, sinews; eyebrows

Positive expressions: Determination, sense of purpose, creativity

Negative emotions: Anger, frustration, repressed anger, rage

Underlying principle

The Wood Element, most active in the spring time of the year, represents growth and awakening. Its nature is expansive, active, and affirmative.

Physical attributes

The major physical signs of Wood are sinewy tendons and a hard body. Wood people either look like tall trees or short, compact bushes. Their strength is in their ligaments, tendons, and sinews. When irritated, they typically clench their fists. They are likely to have dark complexions and broad shoulders. The facial features most strongly related to the Wood Element are the eyebrows and brow bone.

Emotional attributes

Wood types, like green shoots in spring time, have a strong sense of direction and the need to be constantly "doing". They work and play hard. As workers, they can handle tremendous amounts of pressure and strict deadlines. At the same time, like the branches of a tree, Wood types have a tendency to spread themselves too thin in their drive to keep active. Wood people resist aging and fight the weakening of their bodies and try to maintain their high levels of activity both physically and emotionally throughout their lives.

Wood people are very sociable, with good verbal skills and a love of spirited discussion. However, they also tend to have strong tempers, can be quick to take offense, or become frustrated, especially when others don't come through with their obligations. They may have difficulty expressing their innermost feelings.

Wood types have very strong livers and enjoy processing toxins, whether emotional, as caused by anger, or chemical, as in drugs and alcohol. However, failure to process these toxins, for example, hanging on to old anger or resentment, can lead to problems, while too much enjoyment can lead a Wood type to addiction.

Recognizing disharmonies in the Wood Element

>Strong Wood

To keep their natural tendencies in positive expression, Wood types need to pay particular attention to their anger and their need to be active. Their rashness can lead to accidents. They are also prone to injuries of overuse such as strained, pulled or torn muscles and tendons. According to Chinese medical theory, severe cases of overuse of the Wood Element can create conditions like Parkinson's where movement and coordination is compromised and ultimately impeded. Or it can lead to conditions of exhaustion including chronic fatigue. Addiction is another tendency that Wood types need to be aware of, and avoid.

>Stagnant Wood

Stagnant Liver Qi and/or Blood are the most prevalent conditions in people living in modern society. This is the underlying physiological condition associated with impatience and frustration which ultimately lead to such expressions as road rage and aggression. Allowed to develop further, these conditions can implode to depression.

> Deficient Wood

Individuals deficient in the Wood Element may be prone to sudden outbursts of anger, and problems with the nerves, eyes, and tendons, or they may be prone to depression. Menstrual issues in women may also signal Wood Element deficiency.

Achieving harmony in the Wood Element

Green, as the color of the Wood Element, can help overcome a deficient Wood state. Things that you can add to your living environment to support the Wood Element include: constructional materials of wood; tall rectangular shapes, such as a columns or towers; living plants. Sleeping with your head in the east will also increase the influence of Wood.

In terms of diet, the Wood person should avoid eating foods that are greasy and fried. If they notice that they suffer from anger-related issues, then adding sour foods such as lemons, limes, and vinegar to the diet would be very beneficial as the sour flavor stimulates flow of energy in the Liver meridian.

PERSONAL OBSERVATION

It is the nature of Yang to go to excess; the Spring season is at the beginning of the year, when Yang energy is fresh, and just beginning to increase. People of the Wood Archetype, as Wood is the Element of the spring, particularly tend to go to excess. Thus I can often identify a Wood person because they like to have the color green around them everywhere. They will wear green, decorate with green, and even own green cars. This is not always wise, if it exacerbates an already excess situation. However, it is also difficult to tell a Wood person what to do: like those young shoots in spring time, they can be determined and relentless in pursuing their own way.

Chapter 19: THE EMOTIONAL COMPONENT

You have now seen that Chinese medicine recognizes emotional characteristics as symptoms of energetic imbalances. Disease has physical, mental, and emotional aspects; all are both contributing causes and resulting effects. Interestingly, the ancient Chinese texts do not give techniques for specifically addressing emotional imbalances. This is possibly because, in earlier eras, when those texts were written, emotions were not as relatively prominent as they are today. At that time, physical problems were the overriding causes for seeing a doctor. Infectious diseases, accidents, acts of violence, challenges of famine, etc. were the predominant threats to life. Almost no one had a sedentary lifestyle; people had none of the silent stressors that are inescapable aspects of modern life. Instead, most people were farmers, spending time outdoors, alone, as their own boss. Life was certainly not perfect, but it was different.

In today's modern world, as living standards have improved and infectious diseases come under control, emotions have become much more important in the picture of one's overall health. Using the correlations inherent in Chinese medicine's descriptions, we now need to consider both physical and mental symptoms in, or contributions to, any condition. For example, you may have high blood pressure or tinnitus; do you also have anxiety or deep-seated sorrow, or perhaps chronic lack of confidence? To view these as symptoms that you *have* and not qualities that you *are* is important for healing. Modern clinical studies have shown that mental and emotional symptoms can not only generate physical symptoms but also interfere with healing.

Everyone has characteristics; none of them are negative except that thinking makes them so. The natural tendency of the Universe is to create harmony. Allowed to flow freely, energy will find a way to express itself in a positive, healthy way. Whatever your Elemental archetype, whatever your natural inclinations, your natural traits can be transmuted from ore into gold.

How can you identify emotional imbalances? Generally, you can find them in your actions and reactions to stimuli, situations, and people. They are what make you unhappy, resentful, angry, etc. Any negative thought that you have signals an emotional imbalance; when negative thoughts become a persistent internal voice they signal a chronic imbalance—or, in Chinese medicine terms, a place where your energy is stuck. Such phrases as, "I can't stop thinking about…" or "I can't stand…" or "I have never gotten over the loss of…" are all clues to where your energy is not flowing smoothly. When a healthy person gets the flu, he or she suffers until the immune system takes over and restores harmony. Similarly, when a healthy person suffers an emotional loss or stress, he or she suffers--and then recovers. This is the normal process. It's when energy gets stuck that problems arise.

Physical symptoms can also be a clue to underlying problems or unresolved emotional issues. It is the typical chicken-egg conundrum; do physical symptoms cause the mental, or vice versa? This cannot be answered. However the imbalance can be addressed from either side. So, in some cases, physical remedies can resolve emotional issues. This is particularly true of Qigong. For example, when you do the Liver Cleansing Exercise, you may suddenly experience a wave of heat leaving the liver area of the body and flowing downward. What was that? You may never know--and it doesn't matter! The body has just healed itself. Be grateful and move on. Or you may be doing one of the meditations, and suddenly have a new perspective on an old issue, after which the issue is simply no longer important to you. Case closed.

On the other hand, sometimes physical remedies cannot heal the problem. Sometimes they may heal the problem temporarily, but in a day or a week or a month, it comes back, possibly stronger and more intractable than before. Or, sometimes, a remedy will cure the initial problem, but another pops up, possibly worse than the first. Both of these scenarios suggest that the original problem was not actually cured; the disharmony is still there, perhaps transforming, but not dissolving. In this case, a way of addressing the emotional issue directly is needed.

Modern and ancient techniques offer a number of ways to address, heal and harmonize emotional energies. These practices offer important complementary support to Qigong practice in our modern world.

Mindfulness training. This technique has been used for thousands of years to calm the mind. It is derived from the Buddhist practice of Vipassana meditation, now popularized by Jon Kabat-Zinn in books and other publications, and being taught in many clinics and centers around the world. The idea is that you try to keep your mind-attention on the body. That is all. When your mind strays, you bring it back. The key point, however, is to bring it back without frustration, discouragement, or any emotion whatsoever. You simply resume the practice. During the course of this practice, all kinds of thoughts may enter your mind; by patiently discarding them you center the mind in the present moment, in your present body.

NLP, or Neuro-Linguistic Programming. I personally have used this technique with much success. The thrust of the training is to observe how you are distorting actual reality with your mind—to observe how you create negative, self-destructive attitudes that then generate negative, self-destructive actions. Once aware of these patterns, you can change these attitudes, and realize a whole new way of being.

EFT, Emotional Freedom Technique or "Tapping". This is one of the fastest and potentially easiest approaches to resolving emotional issues, requiring no self-discussion or historical analysis. It is based on using Chinese medicine's meridians. The procedure is to hold firmly in mind the negative thought or issue that is plaguing you while you tap vigorously 5-6 times, sequentially, on points on your head and upper torso. The tapping points are actually junctures on acupuncture meridians where emotional energy can get stuck or blocked. Tapping on these points releases the flow of energy. Often what you experience is that a new thought or a new perspective on your situation comes to mind. You then have a choice between the old, painful way of thinking and the new, more balanced, more positive way of thinking. And you will naturally go with the flow into joy. The procedure sometimes has to be repeated because old habits die hard, but the procedure does usually bring immediate as well as long-lasting relief. (The complexities, especially with obstinate cases, are described in books and on websites.)

Mirror talk. Another very simple technique I have used to address emotional issues and create positive change in my life is to talk to myself in the mirror. This may be uncomfortable because it's difficult to face yourself; however, persevere because the practice can bring unexpected benefits.

In addressing emotional issues, talk to yourself in the mirror with compassion and curiosity. Try to find out what is really going on. What is at the root of the problem? Is it fear? Resentment? Jealousy? Your inner self is doing the best that he/she can; simply try to understand. It will seem like you become your higher self talking to your physical self. See what comes up, and allow your higher self to deal with it, keeping in mind your goal of achieving health and harmony.

This technique can also be used to co-create with your higher power (whatever you conceive that to be) positive attributes. In co-creating, there are two important principles to keep in mind. First, always talk and think in terms of the positive. For example if you know you are a controlling person, which is a Liver dysfunction in Chinese medicine, do not say to yourself "Please help me not be a controlling person!" Instead say "I choose to be loving, compassionate, patient, and tolerant!" (or whatever the opposite of controlling is for you). In this way you will always affirm and manifest the positive. Secondly, as you speak to your "self" in the mirror always speak in the present tense. Do not say "I will one day be compassionate," or "I want to be compassionate." Rather, say "I am compassionate!" This is not wishful thinking. In fact you ARE whatever you want to be. The fact that you can conceive of it means that you have the kernel of that quality in yourself; now you want to bring out that quality and let it flourish.

One of my clients recommends continuing this mirror talk until you break into laughter. Laughter is a sure and certain sign of health. Remember, happiness is your natural state.

Self-Reflection Checklist. At the end of this book, in the Appendix, you will find a Self-Reflection Checklist which can further help you address and overcome any negative emotional issues you may have identified, and to help you become a more balanced person. It is a grid, with a list of statements on the left and check-boxes for each day of the month. Read each statement, and then give yourself a red mark if you achieved your goal or a black mark if you did not keep an observance. Do this daily, or as part of your weekly Renewal of Spirit practices. Using the Checklist has two benefits: First, it should make you more aware of negativity that has slipped into your habitual way of being. It is negativity first in thinking, then in action, which creates disease. Second, it shows you the progress that you have made. Acknowledging your progress builds it into your subconscious and promotes further change. At the end of the Checklist are blank lines for you to fill in your own statements. You may like to include some physical symptoms, too. It is odd but true that, as people heal, they forget how sick or dis-eased they used to be. The Self-Reflection Checklist will provide glowing evidence of your progress.

Chapter 20: CONCLUSION

You have now finished the course. You have learned three general meditations for keeping your body in balance: The White Pearl Meditation, the Center & Balance Meditation, and the Micro-Cosmic Orbit. In addition you have learned a physical exercise, and a sound, to harmonize the functions of the Yin organ associated with each of the Five Elements, namely, the Heart, Spleen, Lung, Kidney, and Liver. You are now familiar with Five Element theory and its associations with all the phenomena in the cosmos, from seasons and compass directions to colors and shapes. You have tools to work with the emotional component of your health. In other words you have a firm foundation in understanding how the human being works on an energetic level, and how health is a dynamic balance, affected by emotions, food and your environment. Hopefully, you are also experiencing how the human body is a part of the universe. Qi is expressed in everything.

Your task now is to continue to apply what you have learned: to continue refining your own true nature.

APPENDICES

FIVE ELEMENT CHART

	Fire	Earth	Metal	Water	Wood
Color	Red	Orange	White	Blue	Green
Seasons	Summer	Indian Summer	Autumn	Winter	Spring
Yin Organ (Solid Organs)	Heart Pericardium	Spleen	Lungs	Kidneys	Liver
Yang Organ (Hollow Organs)	Small Intestine Triple Burner	Stomach	Large Intestine	Bladder	Gall Bladder
Negative Emotions	Over Excitation Mania	Anxiety	Sadness Grief	Fear	Anger Rage
Positive Virtue	Love	Balance Fairness Centeredness	Courage	Gentleness Wisdom	Kindness Creativity
Healing Sounds	Hhaaa Shiii	Hhhuuu (who)	SSSSSS	Ffffuuu	Shuuu (shoe)
Tissue	Veins Arteries	Muscles	Hair Skin	Bones	Tendons Ligaments Nerves
Senses	Taste	Touch	Smell	Hearing	Seeing
Orifices	Tongue	Mouth	Nose	Ear	Eyes
Tastes	Bitter	Sweet Bland	Pungent	Salt	Sour
Food Examples	Wine/Port Brandy Coffee/Tea Asparagus Lettuce greens	Honey Sugar Watermelon Fruit Grains	Ginger Onions Garlic Leeks Cinnamon	Kelp Seaweed Seafood	Lemon Plum Pineapple Orange Vinegar

FIVE ELEMENT QUESTIONNAIRE

Instructions:

Below you will find five sections, entitled "Phases", each with a list of questions. For each question, answer how you are, rather than how you want to be. If the question sounds a lot like you, put a +2. If the question sounds somewhat like you, put a +1. Put -1 if not much like you, and a -2 if nothing like you. If you don't know or are unsure, put 0.

When you are done, add up the count for each Phase. Arrange the Phases in order from highest to lowest number. Turn to the Answer page in the Appendix to learn your predominate (highest score) and weakest (lowest score) Element types.

Phase 1:

- Are you a natural born initiator?
- Do you have problems with authority figures?
- Do you suffer from migratory pains?
- Do you act assertively and confidently?
- Does other people's slowness and clumsiness irritate you?
- Do you like struggling against great odds and proving to others you can do it?
- Are you frequently doing something or going somewhere?
- Do you have high blood pressure?
- Have you often been told you do not compromise much?
- Do you always have to be the first and best?
- Does confinement and sitting quietly drive you crazy?
- Do you get frequent muscle cramps?
- Do you like to make the rules and then break them?

- Are you passionate about everything you do?

- Do you pioneer new trails wherever you go?

- Do your nails alternate between hard and thick and dry and brittle?

- Are you impatient with uncommitted people with people with no direction?

- Is your own personal freedom really important in your life?

- Are you afraid to show vulnerability?

- Do you tend to manipulate people and situations to get what you want?

- Is controlling your anger one of your biggest problems?

- Do you find any kind of restraint insufferable?

- Do you do your best work under pressure?

Phase 2

- Would you describe yourself as an introspective "loner"?

- Do you have an exaggerated sex drive?

- Is the search for Truth a prime motivator in your life?

- Do you hate superficiality in people?

- Are you creative, imaginative and original?

- Are you modest and fear being in the limelight?

- Are you self-contained and self-sufficient?

- Is deterioration of teeth and gums a problem?

- Do you seek the deep mystery in everything?

- Are you out of touch with your emotions?

- Do you suffer with backaches frequently?

- Are you tactless and even rude occasionally?

- Do you have a very penetrating and critical mind?

- Is stick-to-activeness one of you strongest virtues?

- Do you have hardening of the arteries?

- Is it hard for you to share with others?

- Do you suffer with isolation and loneliness?

- Are you afraid of losing yourself in others?

- Are you considered enigmatic and eccentric by your friends?

- Do you have remarkable powers of concentration?

- Are you awkward in social circumstances?

- Do you have trouble conforming?

- Have you had kidney or bladder problems?

- Are you watchful and objective with other people?

Phase 3

- Do you spend a lot of time and energy consciously seeking the divine?

- Do you have an enlarged or weak heart?

- Are you charismatic?

- Do you have an extreme aversion to pain?

- Do you love drama, performing and being in the limelight?

- Are you often spontaneous?

- Do you get sores on your tongue and around your mouth?

- Have trouble saying No?

- Do you tend to be more sensual than your friends?

- Have you ever had a speech impediment?

- Do you love to give your opinion?

- Do you fear separation above all else?

- Are you clever on your feet?

- Do you desire fulfillment more than almost anything?

- Do you bore easily with the dull and ordinary?

- Do your cheeks turn red easily?

- Could you be described as extravagant?

- Are you bright and scintillating at social gatherings?

- Do you have eczema?

- Do you have trouble with boundaries?

- Is the need for intimacy a strong motivation with you?

- Does sharing come easily?

- Are you mostly optimistic and enthusiastic about life?

- Are you strongly empathetic?

- Do you suffer from anxiety and insomnia?

Phase 4

- Are you a "law and order" person?

- Do you hold righteousness and virtue in high regard?

- Are rituals important to you?

- Do you have stiff joints and muscles?

- Is chaos your enemy?

- Do you have no time for nonsense?

- Do you hold very precise standards?

- Are you really sensitive to temperature changes?

- Are you intolerant of disorder and dissonance?

- Is your skin and hair really dry?

- Do you fear intimacy?

- Do you have a strong aesthetic sense?

- Does carelessness in others drive you up the wall?

- Are you considered cool, dispassionate, and distant?

- Do you have a tight chest with dry coughing?

- Are reason and high principles your guiding light?

- Are you a little too strict and nit-picky?

- Do you have refined tastes?

- Have you been called self-righteous?

- Do you have a lot of moles and warts?

- Is social involvement on the bottom of your list of important things to do?

- Do you have sinus problems?

- Does your constant self-control drive your spontaneous friends crazy?

- Are you into changing other people?

- Do you suffer from constipation?

Phase 5

- Do you see yourself as a service oriented person?

- Do your friends often use you as a negotiator?

- Is bloating and water retention a problem?

- Do you struggle with inertia and feel "stuck" sometimes?

- Does nurturing come easy to you?

- Are you haunted with self-doubt?

- Do you like to be in charge, but not in the limelight?

- Does your efficiency leave something to be desired?

- Does your need to be accommodating result in conformity?

- Do you often go through an identity crisis?

- Is a need to belong strong in you?

- Do you suffer with muscle tenderness?

- Are you referred to as a "peacemaker" by your friends?

- Do you regard loyalty as being one of the more important traits in a person?

- Are you quite conservative in your thinking?

- Do you have a strong need to be needed?

- Are you often involved in everybody else's business?

- Do you suffer with swollen glands and other lymphatic disorders?

- Would you like things more predictable because things are changing too fast?

- Do you tend to be overly protective?

- Do unrealistic expectations leave you disappointed much of the time?

- Do you try to be all things to all people?

- Is there a deep "emptiness" in the pit of your stomach?

- Do you have a square, solid physique?

FIVE ELEMENT QUESTIONNAIRE ANSWERS

- Phase 1: Wood
- Phase 2: Water
- Phase 3: Fire
- Phase 4: Metal
- Phase 5: Earth

SELF-REFLECTION CHECKLIST

Use the "Self Reflection Check List" at the end of the day. Go through each of these observations. If you did well for the day put a red mark next to the observations and if you did not do well put a black mark. You can add other observations at the bottom if your personal goals or challenges are not included here.

	1	2	3	4	5	6	7	8	9	10	11	12	13	14	15	16	17	18	19	20	21	22	23	24	25	26	27	28	29	30	31
Harming or threatening someone physically or verbally																															
Not trusting others, being suspicious																															
Being unreasonable in making a request																															
Using vulgar language																															
Outwardly expressing my values																															
Feeling depressed when deservedly disgraced																															
Being critical or judgmental																															
Exaggerating, lying, or being deceitful																															
Praising another person																															
Breaking the trust of another person																															
Disgracing another person																															
Being vain, conceited, or acting superior																															

	1	2	3	4	5	6	7	8	9	10	11	12	13	14	15	16	17	18	19	20	21	22	23	24	25	26	27	28	29	30	31
Being overly emotional																															
Being moody																															
Being needy or dependent																															
Being greedy																															
Resenting the success of someone else																															
Holding a grudge																															
Procrastinating																															
Being meddlesome																															
Disrespecting anyone young or old																															
Drinking alcohol																															
Engaging in idle talk or gossip																															
Expressing anger in word or deed																															

	1	2	3	4	5	6	7	8	9	10	11	12	13	14	15	16	17	18	19	20	21	22	23	24	25	26	27	28	29	30	31
Showing patience																															
Being jealous																															
Arguing																															
Complaining about my life, the weather, or the food I eat																															
Seeking revenge																															
Blaming others for my own irresponsibility																															
Holding a prejudice																															
Forgiving someone for their wrongdoing																															
Ignoring a main principle, instead following what's of minor purpose																															
Being late																															

	1	2	3	4	5	6	7	8	9	10	11	12	13	14	15	16	17	18	19	20	21	22	23	24	25	26	27	28	29	30	31
Living in filth																															
Behaving recklessly or irresponsibly																															
Overindulging in anything																															
Doing my best																															
Being lazy																															
Wasting time, money or energy																															
Improper diet																															
Being lazy in my spiritual cultivation																															
Being unorganized																															
Being unreasonable or stubborn																															
Staring at or watching other people																															
Becoming discouraged if I fail to do what I know is right																															

121

RECOMMENDED READING
AND REFERENCES

- *I Ching: The Book of Changes and the Unchanging Truth* by Hua-Ching Ni, Seven Star Communications.

- *The Web That Has No Weaver, Understanding Chinese Medicine* by Ted J. Kaptchuk, O.M.D., Contemporary Publishing Group, Inc.

- *The Foundations of Chinese Medicine, A Comprehensive Text for Acupuncturists and Herbalists* by Giovanni Maciocia, Churchill Livingstone.

- *Face Reading in Chinese Medicine* by Lillian Bridges, Churchill Livingstone.

- Five Element Questionnaire adapted from Mark Johnson

Chris Shelton, MQT

Christopher J. Shelton, M.Q.T. (Medical Qigong Therapist), has the gift of healing. He is known for the remarkable results he achieves with his clients. His passion is to watch people's transformations through the use of Qigong. He started his practice as a healer of the internal arts in 1988, and founded the Morning Crane Healing Arts Center in Willow Glen, CA in 2000. Chris is also a Tai Chi Sifu. He has won many awards including the Grand Championship for the 2010 Tiger Claw Competition. He has been in Kung Fu Magazine numerous times. Due to the outstanding results his clients have experienced he has been interviewed by Showtime, UFC, NBC Sports, San Jose Local TV, Vietnamese TV, and more. When he is not in the clinic Chris enjoys kickboxing, practicing Tai Chi, drawing, and spending time with his family.